1 HOUR MUSCLES

**Give me 1 hour
and I will give you
the muscular physique
you have always
dreamed of.**

No weights, gym or supplements
Fast results in muscle mass
Transform your body

Disclaimer

The information and advice contained in this book are based upon the research and the personal and professional experiences of the author. They are not intended as a substitute for consulting with a health care professional. The publisher and author are not responsible for any adverse effects or consequences resulting from the use of any of the suggestions, preparations, or procedures discussed in this book. All matters pertaining to your physical health should be supervised by a health care professional.

Index

Introduction
This is a basic introduction describing what is
involved in the **1 Hour Muscles** program.

Course Rules
These are a set of rules which you must follow to
make the maximum gains in muscle mass,
fitness and body shape transformation.

Exercises
Here you will learn about the specific exercises
which you will use to transform your body.

Program
Listed here are the exercises which should be
performed in each section of the program.

Keep records of your achievements
Keep photos and measurements to show how
well you have done on this program

Appendix 1 - A-Z of Diets
"Test drive" a variety of diets until
you find one that suits your lifestyle

Appendix 2 - 50 Muscle Building Tips
Some great tips to increase your
muscle mass and strength gains

Introduction

This training manual shows you everything you need to know to achieve a fantastic body shape and fitness levels. It is not bulked up with the usual waffle but gets straight to the point and gives you the information needed to succeed.

All that is required to achieve great results from this manual is your commitment to spend just 20 minutes a day for 3 days a week completing the exercises. **That is just 1 hour per week.** This may not sound like a great deal of time but that is because these exercises are targeted and they will give extremely fast results.

No weights or gym equipment are needed to complete the course which means you can easily train at home without having to visit an expensive gym. Being able to train at home means that you are easily able to fit this course around your existing lifestyle. Even with a lifestyle where you may be away from home on a regular basis, you are still able to complete this program with just 20 minutes in your hotel room.

Another advantage with this course is that it is great for both men and women. Men generally have higher levels of testosterone which build bigger muscles and this is why this course will not give women bulging muscles but will simply give a well toned and strong body whilst keeping a feminine body shape.

There are some course rules which are very important and powerful. You must stick to these rules to achieve maximum results from this course.

The course takes 12 weeks to complete but you will see results soon after starting if you stick to the rules. As your fitness levels improve and your body shape changes, you will feel better and everyone will start to see the physical changes in your body.

Make sure you stick to the program, and to keep yourself motivated, why not keep records of your progress with photographs and taking measurements such as muscle sizes and weight.

Course Rules

These are rules which you must follow to achieve the maximum results. Ignoring these rules will drastically reduce the end result, so you must do your best to keep to the rules.

The only person you are cheating if you ignore the rules will be yourself.

Along with the following rules, I would also recommend that you try to eat a healthy, balanced, low-fat diet while on this course. Try and eat fresh fruit and vegetables, lean meat and low-fat options where possible. You should also drink plenty of water.

Rule 1 - Push yourself to the max

Each exercise must be carried out until you could not manage even one more repetition. You must push each muscle which you are targeting to its limit. If you stop even just one rep before the muscle's maximum, then you are wasting your effort.

Muscles are built up because they are needed to do more work than they are used to. If you stop your exercise before the maximum then your muscles will have no reason to grow.

You should be able to perform around 15 reps of each exercise. If you are completing more reps, you need to increase the intensity of each rep (see Rule 3).

Remember, this is **THE** most important rule
PUSH YOURSELF TO THE MAX

Rule 2 - Rest and relaxation

When muscles are pushed to their max, they need time to repair themselves and build up. This is the reason why exercising is done on alternating days with a full day of rest between each exercise session.

If you start training on a Monday then you should also train on a Wednesday and a Friday with rest days on Tuesday, Thursday and Saturday.

High intensity training methods means that rest is as important as the actual exercises to give the muscles time to grow. Trying to push yourself and over-exercise will actually be harmful to your goals so make sure you get plenty of rest on the days between exercising days to gain maximum results from your efforts.

If you have pushed yourself as hard as you should have done on the exercise days, you will be glad of the rest days anyway as your muscles will be aching as they repair themselves and grow.

Rule 3 - Negative exercising

The title here does not refer to 'bad' exercising. What I mean here is that there are two aspects to moving any weight, there is the lifting of the weight and then there is the lowering (or negative aspect) of the weight. Negative exercising is very important and will greatly improve your results.

The negative aspect of the exercising should take twice as long as the positive aspect. As an example, if you are lifting a weight and it takes 2 seconds, when you lower the weight, it should take 4 seconds.

To increase the intensity of an exercise, you may increase to 4 seconds positive followed by 8 seconds negative.

Take your time with each exercise and do not try to rush them. Make sure you concentrate on the form of the exercise in a smooth movement.

Rule 4 - Consistency

Try and be consistent with your training. If you miss a training session, start that weeks program again.

Make every effort to keep to the same routine when you are exercising so that if mornings are best for you, try and stick to mornings. Humans are creatures of habit, so if you can create a new habit for yourself of exercising in the morning (or afternoon or evening - whichever suits you best) then once you do make it a habit, you will find it easier to stick to it and be consistent.

Another of the advantages of this course is that you do not need any special equipment, so even when you are away from home you are still able to complete the exercises.

NO EXCUSES !

Rule 5 - Targeting

When completing each exercise, you must target the specific muscles for that exercise. Do your best to allow all other un-targeted muscles to be relaxed.

Concentrate on the form of the exercise and you should be able to better target the relevant muscle or muscle group.

Complete the full range of movement for each exercise to make sure that the whole muscle is being fully worked.

Do not try to rush the exercises or you will not be able to target your muscles correctly. Take your time and make sure you are performing the exercise properly to target the correct muscle or muscle group.

Rule 6 - Breathe

This may sound obvious but many people tend to hold their breath when pushing their bodies.

For the exercises to work, your body requires oxygen to produce energy for the muscles. You have to breathe to get this oxygen into your lungs and on to your muscles.

You should be taking your time with your exercises and this will allow you to concentrate and breathe slowly and steadily. There should be no need for you to hold your breath or gasp for air.

Exercises

You will now be taken through all the exercises which will be used in this course. Do not try any of these exercises until you reach the 'Program' section as some of these are for the advanced sections.

Once you have read through the exercise descriptions, you will then be shown the actual program to be followed.

On your 'rest' days, even though you should not complete any of these exercises, I would suggest that you complete some gentle exercising such as long walks, jogging, cycling or swimming. This is not something you have to do but it would help if you are trying to lose fat whilst also building your muscles.

Running on the spot

This is a warm up exercise which will prepare your body for the demands of the exercises and is very important. If you are not warmed up then there is more chance of an injury during exercise. Each 'step' is counted as the left foot on the floor then the right foot on the floor. When that is followed by the left foot on the floor and then the right foot on the floor, that is another 'step'.

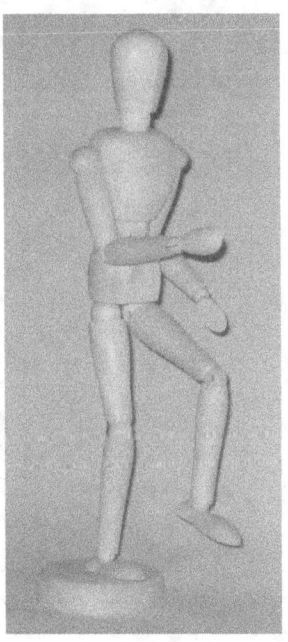

Star Jumps

This is another warm up exercise. Start with your feet together and your hands by your sides. Jump up and land with your feet shoulder width apart and your arms straight and raised to your sides, just above shoulder height (so that you look like a star-fish). Jump again, returning your feet together and your hands back by your sides. This is counted as one star jump.

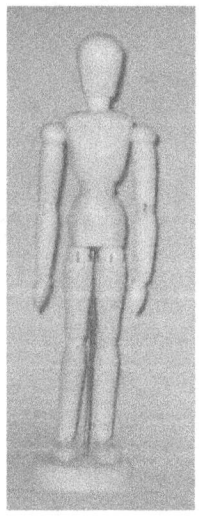 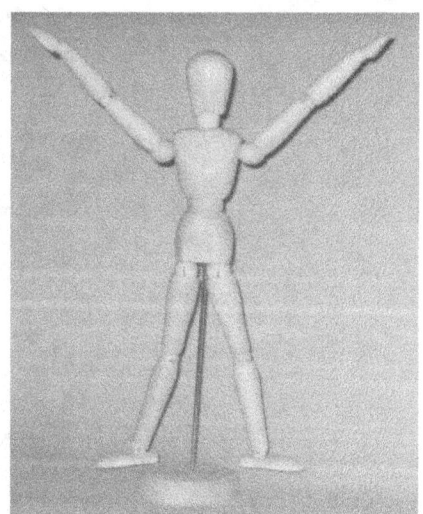

Toe touch stretch

Stand with your feet shoulder width apart. Bend at your waist, keeping your back straight, until your body is parallel to the floor. Twist at your hips and reach to touch your right toes with your left hand while pushing your right arm straight and high into the air behind you. Twist at your hips again to touch your left toes with your right hand while your left arm is pushed straight and high in the air behind you.

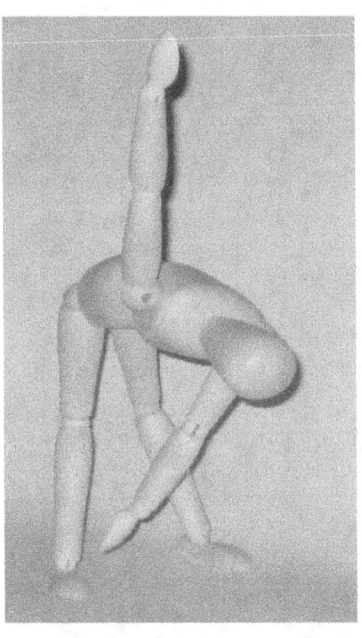

Squat

Start with your feet shoulder width apart. Bend your knees and slowly lower your body. Lean back slightly as you lower yourself down and also roll onto the balls of your feet to allow you to lower yourself further down into a squat position. Briefly pause and then return to the starting position.

The squat is a very important exercise as it is great for overall body conditioning.

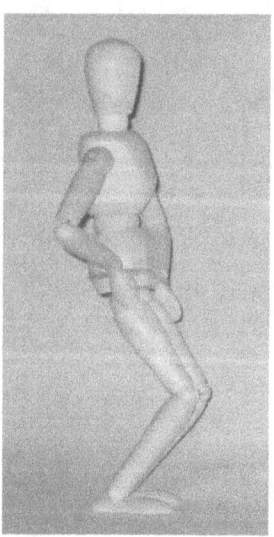

Single leg squat

Stand on a chair or low, solid table with one leg. The other leg should be held slightly to the side so it is out of the way. Bend your knee of the leg you are standing on so that you can lower yourself into a squat position. This is an advanced exercise and you may want to steady yourself by holding onto something and even taking some of the weight with your steadying hand until you are comfortable and confident with this exercise.

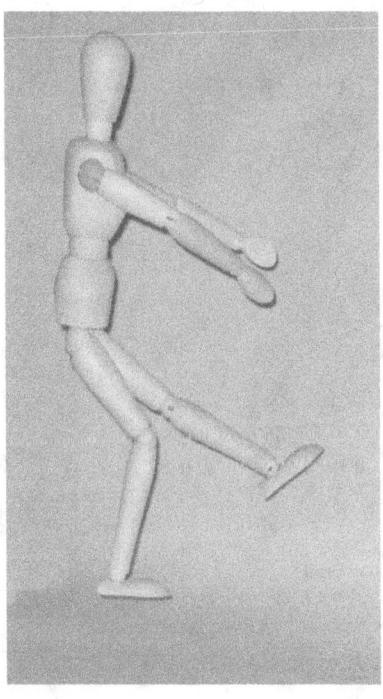

Calf raise

Place something like a thick telephone directory, book or similar on the floor, near a wall. Put the ball of your foot onto the book with the heel of your foot hanging over the edge so that all your weight is on the ball of your foot. Your other leg should be held to the side, out of the way and not allowed to touch the floor.

The book should be thick enough so that you can now lower the heel of your foot down towards the floor but without actually touching the floor. Making sure that you do not bounce, you should now raise your heel into the air, lifting yourself up onto your toes. Lower yourself back down to the starting position and repeat, without letting your heel touch the floor, until you can not manage another rep.

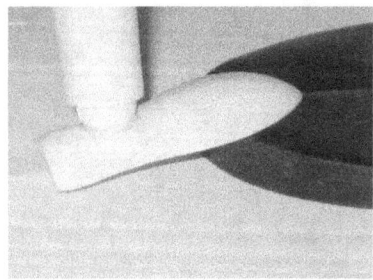 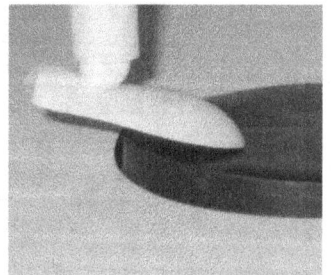

Press Ups

Instead of standard press ups which everyone is aware of, this technique means that you are able to lower your body down further which increases the intensity on your muscles.

Place your hands on to two chairs, either side of your body, with your feet behind you on a third chair. Start with your body straight and straight arms supporting your body weight. Slowly bend your arms at your elbows to lower your body down between the chairs. Lower yourself as far as you can before pushing your body back up to the starting position.

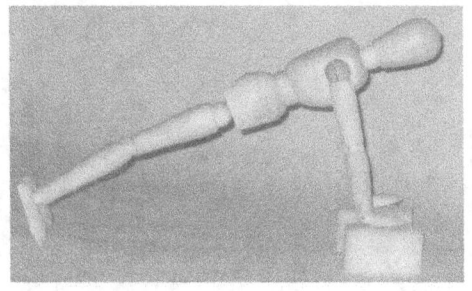

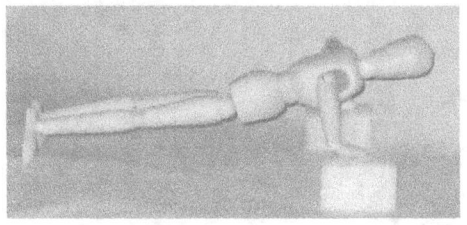

Advanced Press Ups

Place your hands on the floor as you would with the standard press ups but you should place your feet on a chair behind you. This results in more of your bodyweight being placed onto the muscles of your arms.

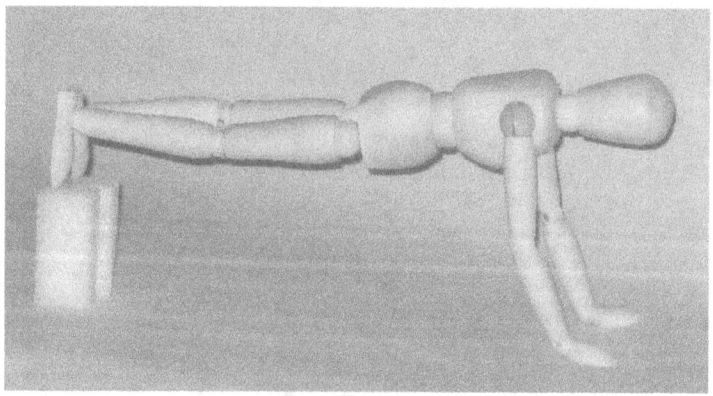

Dips

Support yourself by placing your hands on a chair to the left of you and a chair to the right of you so that you can lower yourself down between the chairs. There should be a third chair in front of you which you should place the heels of your feet on.

Keeping your feet resting on the chair and keeping your legs straight, bend your arms at your elbows to lower your body down between the chairs as far as you can and then raise yourself back up to the starting position.

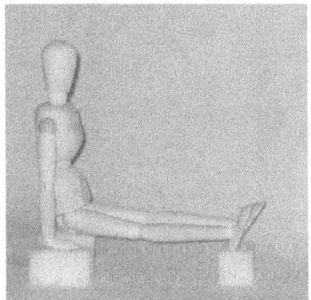 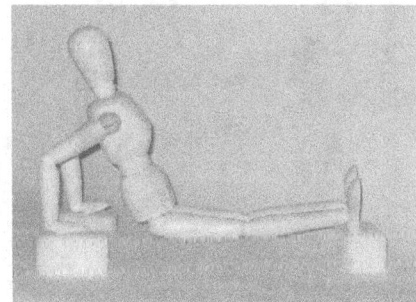

Advanced dips

Support yourself by holding onto the backs of two chairs on either side of you. Bend your knees to lift your legs off the floor. Bend your elbows to lower yourself down as low as you can before raising yourself back to the start position.

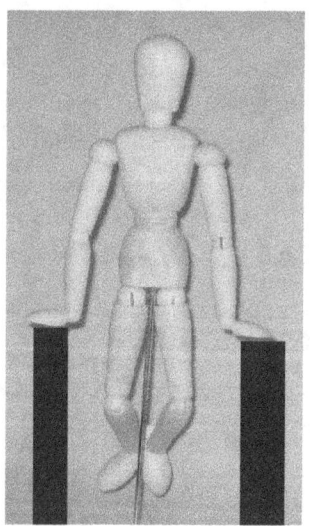 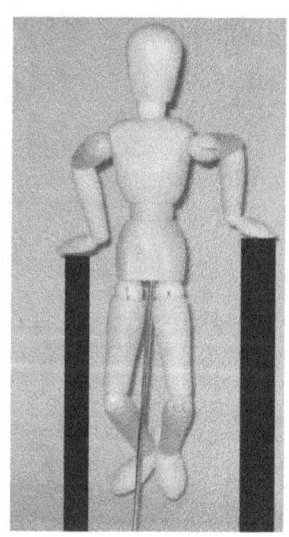

Jack knife

Support yourself by placing your hands on the floor, placed shoulder width apart and about one step distance in front of your feet. Keep your legs together and straight and you should be bent at the waist.

Bend at your elbows to lower your head to the floor and then push yourself back up to the starting position.

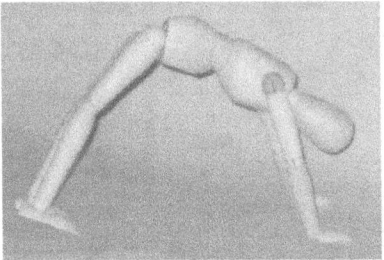 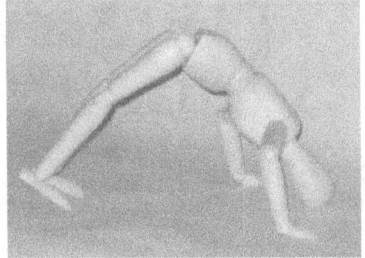

Advanced jack knife

As with the standard jack knife but your feet should be on a chair so that you are raising and lowering more of your body weight.

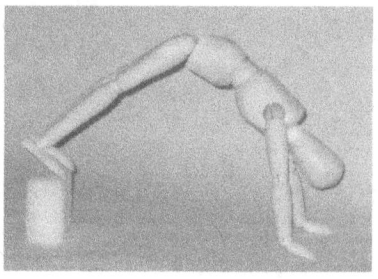 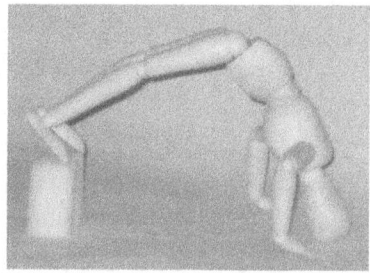

Side laterals

Hold the backs of 2 chairs (or 2 other heavy household items you have to hand) one in each hand and then raise the chairs up to shoulder height, keeping your arms straight, and then lower to about 45 degrees before raising again.

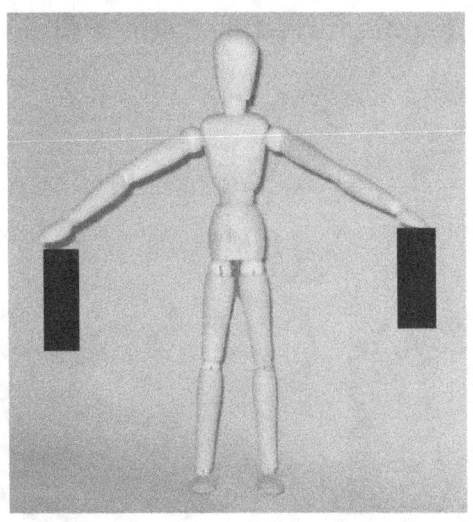

Tricep extensions

Face a wall and stand about one step distance away from the wall. Place your forearms and hands onto the wall (palms against the wall) so that you are leaning onto the wall from your hands down to your elbows. Your hands should be shoulder height with your elbows tucked in towards your body. Keeping your palms on the wall, push yourself backwards to raise your elbows off the wall.

When you have extended your arms, lower yourself slowly back towards the wall until your forearms are resting on the wall again.

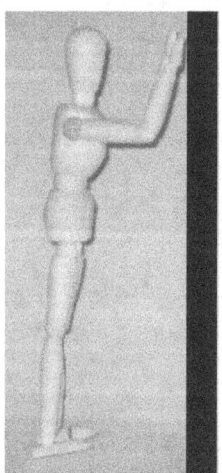 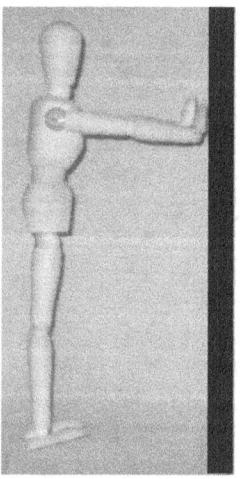

Advanced tricep extensions

Face down on the floor, your forearms and hands should be placed on the floor with your feet raised behind you onto a chair. Keep your body straight and raise yourself off the floor, lifting your forearms off the floor but keeping your elbows tight towards your body.

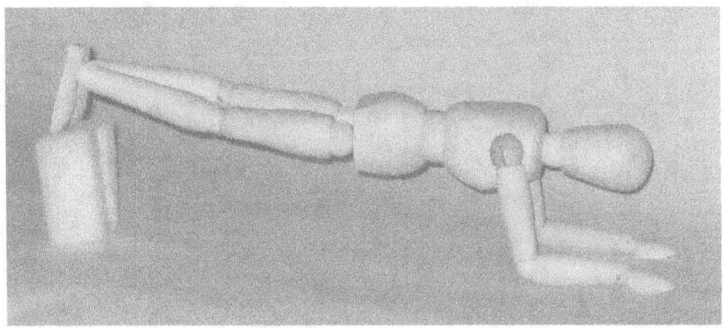

Abdominal crunch

Lie on your back. Bend at your hips to raise your legs off the floor but allow your legs to bend at the knees to lower your feet back down towards the floor, although do not lower your feet to touch the floor as your feet should always be off the floor. Pull your head and shoulders off the floor a few inches. This is the starting position. Crunch your head and knees slightly towards each other and then return to the starting position. Continue sharply crunching your head and knees towards each other.

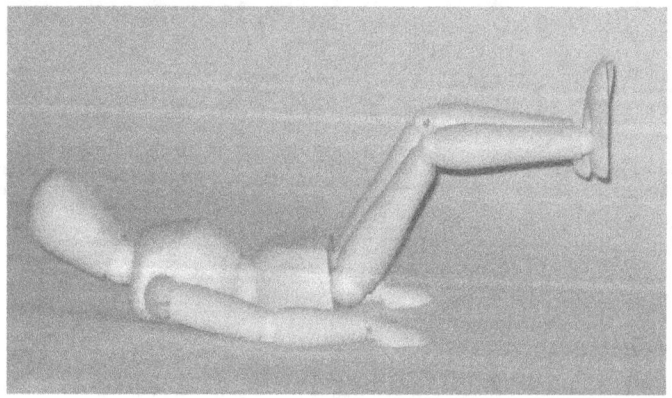

Bicep curls

Find something quite small but heavy although it does not have to be too heavy - a bag of sugar or an ornament would work. Holding the item, with your palms facing upwards, and your elbow held to the side of your body. Bend your arms at your elbows to lift the weight up and down to work your bicep. This can be done without holding an item but by simply tensing your bicep and slowly lifting your fist up and down. Do this action very slowly to really feel the tension.

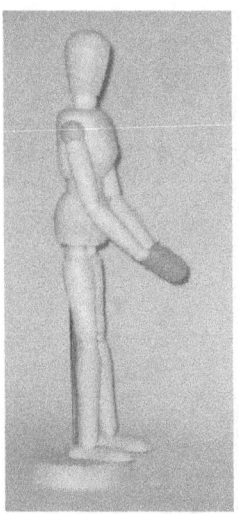 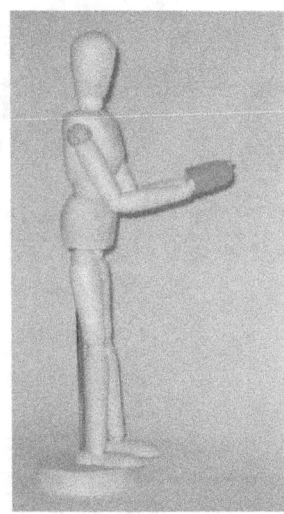

Seated leg raise

Sitting on the edge of a chair with both legs straight out and slightly off the floor. Keeping your legs straight, lift alternate legs as high as you can while keeping the other foot just off the floor.

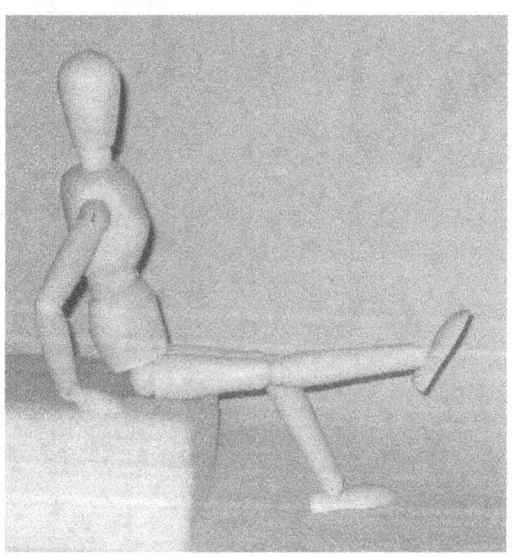

Side bends

Stand up straight with your arms raised straight above your head. Bend at your waist, keeping your arms along the same line as your upper body, first towards your left, return to the upright position and then bend towards your right then back to the upright position. Complete 20 reps.

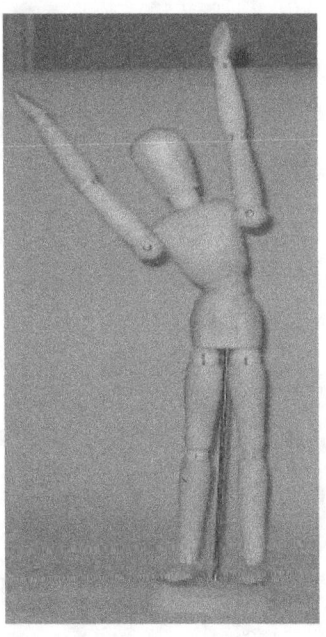

Wrestlers bridge

Warning: Do not perform this exercise to the max. Start with only a few reps at the beginning, working up to a maximum of 20 reps by the end of the program.

Lie on your back with your head on a cushion. Bends your knees and arch your body up off the floor by using your neck muscles. Finish with your feet on the floor and the crown of your head on the cushion with your back arched off the floor. Rock backwards and forwards a couple of times to strengthen your neck muscles.

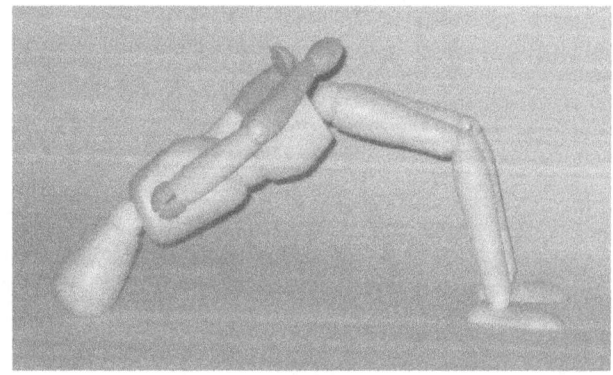

Program

Over the following pages, you will now be given the order in which to complete the exercises over a 12 week period.

The 12 weeks are split up into 4 sections to start you at a beginner level and moving you up towards the most advanced level. Do not skip any of the levels as each one will build upon the previously completed levels.

This is where you take over.

If you put the effort in,
you will be greatly rewarded.

Weeks 1, 2, 3 & 4

Running on the spot (100 steps)

Star jumps (20 jumps)

Squat

Calf Raises

Press ups

Dips

Tricep extensions

Bicep curls

Abdominal crunches

Weeks 5 & 6

Running on the spot (125 steps)

Star jumps (25 jumps)

Toe touch stretch (15 stretches)

Squat

Calf Raises

Press ups

Advanced press ups

Dips

Tricep extensions

Bicep curls

Side Laterals

Seated leg raises

Abdominal crunches

Weeks 7, 8 & 9

Running on the spot (150 steps)

Star jumps (30 jumps)

Toe touch stretch (20 stretches)

Single leg squat

Calf Raises

Press ups

Advanced press ups

Jack knife

Dips

Advanced dips

Tricep extensions

Bicep curls

Side Laterals

Seated leg raises

Side bends

Abdominal crunches

Weeks 10,11 & 12

Running on the spot (150 steps)

Star jumps (30 jumps)

Toe touch stretch (20 stretches)

Single leg squat

Calf Raises

Press ups

Advanced press ups

Advanced jack knife

Dips

Advanced dips

Advanced tricep extensions

Bicep curls

Side Laterals

Wrestlers bridge

Seated leg raises

Side bends

Abdominal crunches

Weeks 12+

To maintain your new physique, continue with week 12 exercises.

If you want to improve even further then you will need to complete multi-sets. Instead of moving straight onto the next exercise, complete an exercise then take 60 seconds maximum rest and then repeat the same exercise. You will not be able to complete as many reps as you did in the first set but you should still push yourself to the max in the second set to achieve as many as you can. Once you have completed 2 sets of the same exercise, you will then move on to the next exercise.

Keep records of your achievements

You may find it useful and motivational to keep records of how much progress you make with this program.

Take photographs of yourself before you start the program along with measurements so that you can compare yourself at different stages. As you look back at how you used to look and compare it with the improvements you have made, it will help to motivate you to keep on with the program.

Take photographs and measurements before you start the program, after 4 weeks, after 9 weeks and after 12 weeks.

Take the following measurements and record them

	Before program	After 4 weeks	After 9 weeks	After 12 weeks
Waist				
Thighs				
Calves				
Forearms				
Biceps				
Chest				
Shoulders				
Neck				

Feedback

Please send your feedback, questions and suggestions to :-
Feedback@1hourmuscles.com

We welcome suggestions for improvements or questions you may have about the 1 Hour Muscles program.

You are welcome to submit reviews to the same email address along with photographs of yourself to show the results which you have achieved from using the program.

Any material submitted to 1HourMuscles.com should be submitted on the basis that 1HourMuscles.com are allowed to use such material, without payment of fees to either party, within future revisions of the 1 Hour Muscles manual or website or associated materials and advertising.

Appendix 1

A-Z of Diets

The A to Z of Diets contains the basics of many different diets and weight loss programs. Giving enough information about each diet should enable you to decide which one suits you and your lifestyle the best.

This book is not meant as a substitute for reading the books which give the full version of the diets, as a more in depth understanding of each diet is required to fully appreciate the concepts and practicalities of each diet. Included in the books explaining the complete diets will be such useful information as meal ideas, facts/figures and diagrams of exercises along with full explanations of the concepts.

Contents

Low Fat

Mayo Clinic

Nutrisystem

Picture Perfect
Dr Phil
Pritikin

Radiant Health Diet

Slim Fast
South Beach Diet
Sugar Busters

Volumetrics

Waterfall Diet
Weight Watchers

Zone Diet

5 Day Miracle Diet

Controlling the body's blood sugar level is the basis for the 5 Day Miracle Diet. Starting the day in low blood sugar, then raising the level by noon and maintaining the level throughout the afternoon and evening will stop cravings for sugary and fatty foods, starches, sweets, alcohol and caffeine. Controlling your blood sugar level also helps with energy levels alleviating lethargy, giving you much more energy but also reduces hyperactivity.

Step 1 - Breakfast
Blood sugar will be low when you wake in the morning and so there is an immediate need to raise the blood sugar to a balanced level. Not correcting your blood sugar level straight away means it will be difficult to correct and creates cravings later in the day. Breakfast should be fast and easy to prepare and consist of a protein and a starch (see Food Choices section). The carbohydrates are quickly broken down to give the body an immediate, quick and necessary rush. The protein is broken down much slower, preventing the crash after the initial blood sugar hit from the carbohydrates.

Step 2 - Hard Chew snack
Eat a hard chew snack (see Food Choices section) within 2 hours of breakfast. This snack can be eaten sooner than 2 hours after breakfast if required but definitely no later than 2 hours. A hard chew snack is a slow release food which will keep your blood sugar level balanced. Examples of the different hard chew snacks are given in the Food Choices section.

Step 3 - Second Hard Chew snack
A second hard chew snack must be eaten within 2 hours of your first hard chew snack. Eating a second hard chew snack within 2 hours of your first will help stabilise blood sugar levels. You must have this second hard chew snack within 2 hours of your first unless you are already eating lunch. If you have breakfast at 8.30am and your first hard chew snack at 10am then you must have your second hard chew snack before 12 noon, even if lunch is only going to be half an hour later.

Step 4 - Lunch
Lunch should not be eaten any later than 1pm and should include protein and vegetables. A small amount of hard chew vegetables should also be included in your lunch. Blood sugar is now stabilised and should be kept balanced for the rest of the day.

Two rules which you must adhere to are:-
(i) You can not save bread for the evening meal as metabolism is slower in the evening and calories eaten at night stay on the body.
(ii) Never eat pasta at lunch and limit pasta to only twice a week. Pasta is too glycemic meaning that it is too easily broken down creating drowsiness and cravings.

Step 5 - Afternoon snacks
During the afternoon you must eat one or two more snacks but they must be spaced no more than 3 hours apart. Now that the blood sugar level is controlled, the snacks can be either hard or soft chew as you now only have to maintain blood sugar rather than create it. If the time between your lunch and dinner is more than 6 hours then you should make sure you have two snacks between the meals otherwise harmful foods become much too tempting as blood sugar levels drop and you start to have cravings.

Step 6 - Dinner

Try to eat dinner no later than 8pm and earlier if possible. Dinner should consist of vegetables and protein. The vegetables can be cooked to have a soft chew texture as it is not necessary to have hard chew at night. If there was no starch with lunch you can have it now with dinner but bread is a lunchtime option only and may not be saved for dinner. However, bread may be included for dinner in place of the carbohydrate choice.

Emergency Quick Fixes

Grab these when the craving just will not stop. They supply the sweetness a craving wants but holds the craving back until it disappears. See the Food Choices section for a list of emergency quick fixes.

Exercise

Exercising is an important part in your weight loss success but try stabilising your blood sugar level first. After 5 days of stabilising your blood sugar you will have so much more energy than before that you will want to exercise. Just think about taking the stairs rather than the escalator, getting off the bus a few stops early and think about walking instead of taking the car.

A Few Rules

Listed below are a few rules to follow which will further help with your weight loss and also increase the health benefits.

(i) Drink 8 glasses of water a day
(ii) Take a multi-vitamin and mineral supplement at breakfast
(iii) Take a calcium pill at bedtime
(iv) It is fine to use fat - but use it sparingly
(v) Limit salt

Food Choices

Hard Chews:

2 carrots
10 baby carrots
1 cup of string beans
1 baby cucumber
2 stalks of celery
1 medium apple
1 medium pear
4 asparagus stalks

Soft Chews:

1 medium peach
2 small plums
1/2 grapefruit
4 small apricots
1 medium orange
100g strawberries

60g blueberries
1 medium nectarine

Emergency Quick Fix:
1 slice cantaloupe melon
1/4 orange
1/2 unsalted pretzel
1/2 slice wholegrain bread
1 apple
1 pear
Herbal tea

Typical Breakfast Choices
Women - lower portion amounts   Men - higher portion amounts

Protein:
You can mix and match your choices but do not exceed the noted amounts. For example, you can have 1 slice of cheese and 1 egg.
2-3 egg whites
1 egg yolk and 2 egg whites
90-110g tofu
2-3 teaspoons peanut butter
2 slices low fat cheese
30-60g tuna or salmon
30-60g hard cheese

Starchy Carbohydrates:
1 slice wholegrain bread
2 rice cakes
1 slice rye bread

Typical Lunch & Dinner Choices:
Women - lower portion amounts   Men - higher portion amounts

Protein:
You can mix and match your choices but do not exceed the noted amounts. For example, you can have 60g tuna and 80g skinless chicken.
1-2 eggs
2 egg whites and 1 yolk
90-150g low fat cheese
30-60g hard cheese
60-140g tuna or salmon
60-140g skinless chicken
110-140g tofu
60g-140g shell fish
60-140g lean beef, pork or lamb

Vegetables:

Any variety of non-starchy vegetables either steamed, grilled, stir-fried or raw in a salad. Eat at least 2 servings of vegetables at dinner.

Starchy Carbohydrates:
At dinner or lunch, every day for men, alternate days for women.
1 medium baked potato
70-150g brown rice
60-110g pasta (at dinner only)
80-110g peas
70-150g barley or other grains
70-150g couscous
100-150g beans

7x7 Fat-Reducing Plan

The new 7x7 Fat-Reducing Plan is successful, safe and extremely easy to follow. The diet works on the principles followed by many Asian cultures with populations that are lean and disease-free. It also recognises recent breakthroughs made by scientific studies on reducing the 'energy density' of our food. By following the plan you will not overeat, allowing your body easier access to your fat stores. But you will not go hungry, either.

The Seven-Day Plan

Seven meals a day seems like a bit of a tall order, you may think, but it is the way forward in effective fat stripping. Cultures that exhibit very good health as well as good weight control don't gorge or eat to full capacity. The emphasis is on grazing. I spent over a year living in Italy, where I found that eating several small meals a day is quite normal. You may even have four courses in one meal but the amounts are always small, as in this plan.
The aim of the 7x7 Fat-Reducing Plan is to:
Eat less food more often, so as not to overeat or eat in between meals
- Keep fat intake down
- Increase fibre intake
- Reduce the amount of energy we eat
- Consume enough nutrients
- Lose body fat

The focus of the eating plan is to keep fat intake to a minimum, thus allowing your body to use its own fat stores for energy, and to increase fibre intake. It breaks your food into much smaller meals and speeds up your metabolism. The faster you burn this food up, the faster your metabolism will be, and the faster you will burn fat. One of the keys to success is to include vegetables or salad with every evening meal. You must eat these first and finish them before you eat the rest of your meal.

Monday
Breakfast
1 high-fibre muffin, with a scraping of margarine and Vegemite
1 glass of orange juice
Mid-morning snack
1 banana
1 orange or other fruit
Lunch
½ - 1 pitta bread with salad & ham
2 glasses of water
Mid-afternoon snack
1 small tub of low-fat yoghurt
Late-afternoon snack
1 apple
Dinner
Large bowl of homemade vegetable soup with 2 pieces of bread
1 glass of water
Dessert
Fresh fruit salad

Tuesday
Breakfast
Small bowl of oats, with low-fat milk
1 glass of orange juice
Mid-morning snack
1 banana
1 orange or other fruit
Lunch
Bowl of spicy broth with 1-2 pieces of bread
2 glasses of water
Mid-afternoon snack
1 slice of fruit bread
Late-afternoon snack
1 small tub of low-fat yoghurt
1 mandarin
Dinner
2 servings of pulses, such as chickpeas and lentils, with rice
1 glass of water
Dessert
1 small scoop of low-fat ice cream

Wednesday
Breakfast
2 pieces of fruit bread, with a scraping of margarine and strawberry jam
1 glass of orange juice
Mid-morning snack
1 banana
1 orange or other fruit
Lunch
Low-fat Caesar salad with 1-2 pieces of bread
2 glasses of water
Mid-afternoon snack
1 pear or other fruit option
Late-afternoon snack
1 muesli bar
Dinner
1 small bowl of pasta, with seafood or lean mince sauce, with salad
1 glass of water
Dessert
Fresh fruit platter

Thursday
Breakfast
1 small bowl of low-fat cereal, with low-fat milk and fruit
1 glass of orange juice
Mid-morning snack
1 banana

1 orange or other fruit
Lunch
1 salmon and salad sandwich or roll
2 glasses of water
Mid-afternoon snack
1 muesli bar
Late-afternoon snack
1 small tub of low-fat yoghurt
Dinner
A small piece of lean beef, and 2 different serving of pulses, with vegetables and rice
1 glass of water
Dessert
1 small scoop of gelati (low-fat Italian ice cream)

Friday
Breakfast
2 pieces of wholemeal toast, with a scraping of margarine and jam
1 glass of orange juice
Mid-morning snack
1 banana
1 orange or other fruit
Lunch
½ - 1 pitta bread with roast beef and salad
2 glasses of water
Mid-afternoon snack
1 apple or other fruit
Late-afternoon snack
1 muesli bar
Dinner
Grilled or baked fish or chicken with steamed vegetables or a small bowl of pasta with a tomato-based sauce and salad
1 glass of red wine
Dessert
Fresh fruit platter

Saturday
Breakfast
Banana smoothie, made with low-fat milk
Mid-morning snack
1 banana
1 orange or other fruit
Lunch
1 tuna and salad sandwich or roll
2 glasses of water
Mid-afternoon snack
4-5 rice crackers with low-fat tzatziki dip
Late-afternoon snack
1 small tub of low-fat yoghurt

1 orange
Dinner
Grilled or baked fish with steamed vegetables, or a small bowl of pasta with a tomato-based sauce and salad
1 glass of red wine and 1 glass of water
Dessert
1 small scoop of low-fat frozen yoghurt

Sunday
Breakfast
2 Weetabix, with low-fat milk
1 glass of orange juice
Mid-morning snack
1 banana
1 orange or other fruit
Lunch
Your choice (but not chips!)
Mid-afternoon snack
1 small tub of low-fat yoghurt
Late-afternoon snack
1 muesli bar
1 apple
Dinner
Your choice (be sensible!)
Dessert
Your choice

As you can see, the plan does not dictate seven large meals that will have you bursting at the seams, nor are there complicated ratios of foods that require hours to prepare. Instead, there are seven opportunities to eat during the day.

Fish has been included regularly on the menu, but if you dislike fish, take some fish oil supplements every two or three days. Remember: fish oil taken in recommended amounts doesn't get converted into fat but rather into hormones that are involved in regulating your blood pressure.

The 7x7 Fat-Reducing Plan includes a variety of pulses such as red kidney beans and lentils. These foods promote healthy fat loss. It's important to try to include some in this eating plan once or twice a week. Include vegetable soup, with plenty of different coloured vegetables, at least once or twice a week.

Abs Diet

Just can't get rid of your flabby belly, even though you do sit-ups and crunches until you're ready to drop? Maybe you're so mortified by the condition of your abs that you've relegated your bikini and low-rise jeans to the dark recesses of your closet.

Before you dump on (or just plain dump) your workout for not giving you killer abs, you should know the real culprit may be your diet -- or even your high-stress lifestyle.

If you want to go from fat to fab abs, new research shows that what you eat is just as important as how -- or even how much -- you work out. And lifestyle counts, too, because stress doesn't just mess with your head, it also can induce a pooch.

Following are six strategies from the country's leading weight-loss, nutrition and stress experts, all designed to get you flat abs in just four weeks, plus three delicious, low fat recipes that will fill you up without making you look or feel bloated.

6 steps to flatter abs

Tip 1. Eat more fibre.
Not eating enough fibre may be a major reason women are getting fatter and flabbier. To ditch the fat and show off firm, beautiful abs, you need to eat at least 25 grams of fibre daily, says leading fibre researcher David J.A. Jenkins, M.D., Ph.D., D.Sc., professor of nutrition at the University of Toronto, and a member of the National Academy of Sciences (NAS) Food and Nutrition Board. Fibre, which is the indigestible part of fruits, vegetables and whole-grain foods, helps you achieve flat abs for three reasons:

The "bulk" factor Fibre is like a dry sponge. When it combines with the water in your digestive tract, it makes everything move through more quickly.

The "fill" factor Because high-fibre foods like fruits and vegetables supply plenty of bulk to your meals without adding a lot of calories, they keep you feeling full longer and help you lose weight, according to a study at the Human Nutrition Research Centre at Tufts University. Researchers concluded that low fat diets work only if they're also high in fibre-rich foods like fruits, vegetables and whole grains, all of which fill you up on fewer calories and less fat. In contrast, low fat diets that are low in fibre and high in sugar, salt and preservatives can lead to bloating and weight gain.

In a study conducted by Barbara Rolls, Ph.D., a professor at Penn State University and co-author of The Volumetrics Weight-Control Plan (HarperTorch, 2003), subjects who ate vegetables as part of their meals consumed about 100 fewer calories and didn't make up for the caloric deficit later. While saving 100 calories a day may not sound like much, it translates into losing 10 pounds in one year. Use just this one trick -- and there goes your tummy!

The "chew" factor "High-fibre foods require more chewing and take longer to eat," explains Leslie Bonci, M.P.H,, R.D., author of the American Dietetic Association Guide to Better Digestion (John Wiley & Sons, 2003). "Because your mouth is more involved in the eating of high-fibre foods, you feel more satisfied with a high-fibre meal."

How to add fibre to your diet comfortably One cautionary note: It's important to add fibre slowly but consistently to prevent gas. "Make higher-fibre choices throughout the day; don't have all your fibre in one bunch," Jenkins says. "This is particularly important with viscous fibre -- a type of soluble fibre found in beans, oats and barley that also has the benefit of lowering blood cholesterol," he says.

For best results, increase your fibre intake slowly over the course of one month and drink plenty of water to keep food moving through your system as quickly as possible.

Tip 2. Opt for a sensible amount of high-quality carbs.
For flatter abs, make carbs 45-65 percent (202-292 grams based on an 1,800-calorie diet) of your total daily calories. Balance is the key here, so don't go below 45 percent (202 grams), or above 65 percent (292 grams), which can lead to water retention, bloating and temporary weight gain that shows up in your middle.

When you eat carbs, they break down into glucose, which is stored as glycogen in the muscles and liver. When glycogen is stored, it carries with it three times its own weight as water, compared to no water at all for protein and fat, according to Peter Garlick, Ph.D., a professor at Stony Brook University in New York. If you eat an extremely high-carb diet, you may store excess water, experience bloating and gain temporary water weight. (This is why people who go on no- or very low-carb diets can initially lose weight so quickly. They're really just losing water.)

To avoid bloating and weight gain caused by consuming too many or the wrong kind of carbs, follow these tips:
* Fill up on fruits and vegetables. These are the least bloat-promoting foods because they contain plenty of water and fewer carbs and calories for their volume.
* Avoid high-carb/empty-calorie foods like fast food, snack cakes, cookies and candy. These foods are high in simple carbs and sodium, which cause bloating and weight gain, and are low in fibre and nutrients.
* Focus on balanced eating. For best results, eat at least three to five 4-ounce servings of veggies (15-25 grams of carbs); two to four 4-ounce servings of fruit (30-60 grams of carbs) and about 1 cup (8 ounces cooked or 2 ounces dry, or 2 slices of bread) of whole grains per meal (90 grams per day).
* Make sure you eat enough calories, from complex carbs, lean protein and healthy fats. If you don't get an adequate number of calories (most women require at least 1,800 per day to lose weight, 2,000 to maintain and 2,400 or more if they're very active), you risk temporarily lowering your metabolism, which can also bring on bloating.

A good guideline: Don't cut any more than 250-500 calories below what you need to maintain your weight, advises C. Wayne Callaway, M.D., a metabolic specialist in Washington, D.C.

Tip 3. Drink up!
Many women believe that drinking too much water will give them puffy abs, but just the opposite is true. 'Even though we associate water with being bloated, drinking more water can help to flush sodium out of the body, and that reduces the bloat," said Jeff Hampl, Ph.D., R.D., nutrition researcher and assistant professor at Arizona State University.

Flat Abs Recipes

Now that you've got the perfect tips for flatter abs, you need the perfect meals to go with them. Each dish here is crammed with fibre so you'll benefit from the bulk, fill and chew factors.

Every recipe also has a good balance of carbs, protein and fat. Check out the low sodium numbers, which are right where you need them to be to prevent bloating, as well as the calorie counts, and make sure you choose your leanest meal at night, when calories should be their lowest.

Blueberry-Banana Pancakes Serves 4

Prep time: 10 minutes
Cook time: 10-15 minutes

Nutrient note A great beginning to your day -- whole-wheat flour is a good source of fibre and B vitamins, blueberries contain powerful antioxidants, bananas are rich in potassium, and milk is chock-full of calcium. Non-stick cooking spray

1 cup whole-wheat flour
1/2 cup all-purpose flour
2 tablespoons sugar
2 teaspoons baking powder
1/4 teaspoon salt
3 very ripe medium bananas
1 cup non-fat milk
1 egg
1 teaspoon vanilla extract
1 1/2 cups frozen blueberries (do not defrost)
4 tablespoons maple syrup

Preheat oven to 250[degrees] F. Coat a griddle or large non-stick skillet with cooking spray and preheat.

In a medium bowl, combine both flours, sugar, baking powder and salt. Mix well with a fork and set aside.

In a large bowl or food processor, mash bananas until mushy. Add milk, egg and vanilla and mix or process until blended.

Add dry ingredients to banana mixture and mix or process until just blended (tiny lumps should still appear; do not over mix or pancakes will be tough). Ladle 3 tablespoons of batter onto hot griddle for each pancake. Top each with 1-2 tablespoons of blueberries.

When bubbles appear around the edges of pancakes, after about 2-3 minutes, flip and cook 1 minute. Transfer pancakes to a warm plate and keep warm in a 2500 F oven while you cook remaining pancakes.

Serve pancakes with maple syrup over top.

Nutrition Score per serving (3 pancakes plus? tablespoon maple syrup): 384 calories, 6% fat (3 g;

<1 g saturated), 83% carbs (80 q), 11% protein (11 g), 8 g fibre, 203 mg calcium, 3 mg iron, 401 mg sodium.

Chicken Fried Rice Serves 4
With Vegetables

Prep time: 10 minutes
Cook time: 40 minutes

Nutrient note This lightened-up Asian classic combines skinless chicken, an excellent source of high-quality protein, with brown rice (a good source of fibre), carrots (loaded with beta carotene), peas (crammed with folate) and green onions (full of cancer-fighting sulphur compounds).

2 teaspoons sesame oil
1/2 cup chopped onion
2 garlic cloves, minced
1 pound skinless, boneless chicken breasts, cut into 1/2-inch pieces
1 cup uncooked brown rice
1 tablespoon reduced-sodium soy sauce
1 cup diced carrots
2 1/4 cups reduced-sodium chicken broth
1/2 teaspoon salt
1/4 teaspoon ground black pepper
1/4 cup frozen green peas, thawed
1/4 cup chopped green onions

Heat oil in a medium saucepan over medium heat. Add onion and garlic and saute 2 minutes, until soft. Place chicken in saucepan and saute 5 minutes, until browned on all sides, stirring frequently. Add rice and cook 1 minute, until translucent. Stir in soy sauce to coat rice.

Add carrots, chicken broth, salt and pepper and bring mixture to a boil. Reduce heat, cover and simmer 30 minutes, until liquid is absorbed and rice is tender.
Stir in peas and green onions and heat through.

Nutrition Score (1[1/2] cups):375 calories, 17% fat (7 g; 1.5 g saturated), 47% carbs (44 g), 36% protein (34 g), 4 g fibre, 42 mg calcium, 2 mg iron, 781 mg sodium.

Grilled Vegetables and Hummus on Whole-Grain Baguette

Serves 4
Prep time: 10 minutes
Cook time: 6 minutes

Nutrient note This excellent lunch boasts eggplant, a good source of protein, potassium and calcium; zucchini, which serves up folate; tomatoes and red peppers, which boast vitamin C; hummus, which contains a fair amount of protein; and whole-grain bread, which dishes up fibre and B vitamins.

Olive-oil cooking spray

2 small eggplants (about 1/2 pound total), cut lengthwise into 1/4-inch-thick slices
1 medium zucchini (about 1/2 pound), out lengthwise into
1/4-inch-thick slices
1 beefsteak tomato, sliced into
1/4-inch-thick slices
Salt and ground black pepper
1/2 cup prepared hummus
2 roasted red peppers, from water-packed jar, thinly sliced
1 cup fresh basil leaves
1 8-ounce whole-grain baguette, halved horizontally

Preheat outdoor grill, stovetop grill pan or broiler.

Spray both sides of eggplant, zucchini and tomato slices with olive-oil spray and season with salt and black pepper to taste. Grill or broil eggplant, zucchini and tomato slices 3 minutes per side, until golden brown and tender.

Spread hummus on one half of baguette. Top hummus with grilled vegetables and then roasted red pepper slices and basil leaves. Top with second half of bread to make a sandwich. Slice baguette into 4 equal sandwiches and serve.

Nutrition Score per serving (1 sandwich): 200 calories, 14% fat (3 g; <1 g saturated), 68% carbs (34 g), 18% protein (9 g), 10g fibre, 190 mg calcium, 3mg iron, 188mg sodium.

An easy way to tell if you're drinking enough is by checking the colour and quantity of your urine. If it's pale yellow and high volume, you're doing OK. If it's dark and scant and/or you're thirsty, you're very likely to be dehydrated.

Follow these tips to stay hydrated and healthy:
* Drink at least eight 8-ounce glasses of water per day. Beverages with little or no calories, caffeine or sodium, including herbal tea, are best. Avoid regular soft drinks and soups with lots of sodium. If you are eating plenty of water-rich foods such as fruits, vegetables and low-sodium soups, you can get half of your water requirements from foods, according to a 1998 NAS Food and Nutrition Board report.

* Avoid carbonated drinks. Fizzy drinks, including soda pop and spritzers, increase bloating because the carbon dioxide trapped in the bubbles creates gas, which slows down stomach emptying.
* Watch your intake of alcohol and caffeine. Both are natural diuretics, which increase fluid loss and don't replace your body fluids as effectively as water, juice and caffeine- and alcohol-free beverages. Because they promote dehydration, alcohol and caffeine also can fatten abs.

Tip 4. Watch the sodium.
Sodium may have a bad rep, but it's essential for regulating body fluids and blood pressure as well as for nerve transmission, muscle function and absorption of important nutrients. But even a small amount of excess sodium causes bloating.

According to the NAS, the average woman needs only 500 milligrams of sodium a day. Most of us get more than six times that, or 3,000-6,000 milligrams per day. The consequence of all this sodium -- most of which is consumed as salt and preservatives in processed foods, fast foods and restaurant foods -- isn't pretty for your abs. That's because where sodium goes, water follows.

When you eat a high-sodium meal, say, from your favourite Chinese takeout at 3,000 milligrams per entree, your body responds by retaining water. This results in edema and, possibly, a rise in blood pressure. Sodium's visible traces are outlined the next day when you stand sideways in your full-length mirror: major B-L-O-A-T! Even though it's temporary, that's no consolation when you Want to wear something revealing that day.

Here's how to keep your sodium intake at a healthy level:
* The American Heart Association recommends you consume no more than 2,400 milligrams of sodium daily -- roughly 1 teaspoon of table salt. That's enough sodium to replenish your supply even if you work up a major sweat.
* Choose fresh, natural foods over fast, commercial or packaged foods. Instead of ordering French fries (265 milligrams of sodium), have a baked potato (8 milligrams). Instead of a pickle (1,730 milligrams!), enjoy a fresh cucumber (6 milligrams). And beware of cured meats: Three ounces of ham packs in 1,009 milligrams of sodium. compared to just 48 milligrams for the same amount of roast pork. Soups are also notoriously high in sodium; some canned varieties contain more than 1,100 milligrams per cup. Read labels carefully and stick with low-sodium brands like Healthy Choice.

Tip 5. Eat light at night.
It never fails: You have a heavier-than-normal evening meal or snack, and When you weigh yourself the next morning, you're up by several pounds. But as depressing as it may seem at the moment, such a quick gain is always water weight; you simply cannot gain that much fat overnight.

Evening eating is often the most problematic for women, as it can be related more to emotional issues than to real hunger. You're tired, lonely, bored, anxious; you want to relax or reward yourself after a tough day. But indulge too many nights in a row and that temporary water gain becomes permanent fat gain -- and fatter abs.
In a study conducted by Callaway, people who skipped breakfast or lunch and ate their largest meal later in the day had lower metabolisms. So by eating light at night you'll receive a double benefit: You'll wake up with a flatter tummy, and you'll also have a better appetite for a fibre-rich breakfast, which sets you up for a day of healthful eating.

Some tips to get you started:
* Eat five times a day. Your body needs food every three to four hours, so instead of eating three large meals, try to schedule five smaller, more frequent meals throughout the day (breakfast-snack-lunch-snack-dinner). By staying full and energized, you'll avoid hunger pangs, maintain an even energy flow, make better, healthier food choices (no bingeing or craving) and enjoy the most efficient burning of calories.
* Eat two-thirds of your calories before dinner. Your body needs calories when you're active, not at night, when your natural rhythm is slowing down. Make sure to eat breakfast, lunch and dinner to keep your metabolism revved.
* If you have to eat at night because you're hungry, stick with fruit, vegetables and other foods that are low in fat, calories and sodium.

Tip 6. Reduce stress.

Research shows that stress triggers the hormone cortisol to turn up your appetite and deposit fat around the organs in your abdomen. Pamela Peeke, M.D., M.P.H., author of Fight Fat After Forty (Penguin, 2000) calls this "toxic weight," because it's associated with heart disease, diabetes and cancer.

"Worrying over an issue that will not go away can lead to prolonged increases in your cortisol," says Peeke. "That means one heck of a stress-related appetite and fat abs."

To reduce stress-related eating, try these tips:
* Move it to lose it. A recent study conducted at the Fred Hutchinson Cancer Research Centre in Seattle showed cardiovascular exercise is especially effective in reducing midsection weight gain.
* Chill out. When you feel stress building, take a few moments to breathe deeply and regroup.

RELATED ARTICLE: 4 tips for bikini abs
* Eat lots of fibre and complex carbs - they'll keep you feeling full longer and aid in weight loss.
* Drink at least eight glasses of water daily to speed digestion. Aerobic exercise will whittle your middle, so hit the beach and get moving!
* Eat fruit to satisfy your sweet tooth and take the edge off your appetite.

4-week fibre-up guide
Here's a four-week guide on how to up your fibre intake without uncomfortable side effects. Each week you'll add a fibre-rich option to one more of your meals, gradually building to 24-27 grams of fibre every day.

Week 1 Every morning, supplement your favourite breakfast cereal with 1/4 cup of General Mills Fibre One (adds 7 grams of fibre). Enjoy one piece of fresh fruit too (adds 2-3 grams of fibre). * Fibre tally: 9-10 grams daily
Week 2 For lunch, make a sandwich using 100 percent whole-wheat bread (adds 4 grams of fibre). Plus, have 1 cup of raw vegetables (adds 2 grams of fibre). * Fibre tally: 15-16 grams daily

Week 3 For dinner, sprinkle 1/4 cup garbanzo, pinto or black beans on a salad, soup or stew (adds 3 grams of fibre). As a side dish, eat 1/2 cup sautéed dark leafy greens (adds 2 grams of fibre). * Fibre tally: 20-21 grams daily

Week 4 Every day, snack on a piece of fruit midmorning and then again in the afternoon (adds 4-6 grams of fibre). * Fibre tally: 24-27 grams daily

Atkins Diet

The Atkins Diet was launched in the 70's when Dr. Atkins published the New Diet Revolution. Atkins spoke up against the medical establishment and told us of the effects of sugar and carbs in foods, and how managing your intake of carbs would lead to weight loss.

The two week induction phase of the Atkins Diet is the strictest phase of the diet, where only pure proteins are allowed, and a very limited amount of carbs. The proteins allowed include meat, fish, poultry, and eggs, an pure fats such as olive oil, butter, and mayonnaise.

Only 20 grams of carbohydrates per day are allowed during this period, via vegetables such as broccoli, salad, and asparagus. No bread, grains, starchy vegetables or fruit should be eaten during this phase.

The dieter then moves through two more phases, slowly building their carbohydrate intake, until they know how much can be eaten without putting on weight - and moves into the Life time maintenance phase.

The Atkins Diet Plan is made up of 4 phases. The induction phase, on going weight loss, pre-maintenance and lifetime maintenance.

Induction
The purpose of the first 2 weeks induction phase of the Atkins diet, as written in the Dr Atkins New Diet Revolution, is to start a change in you metabolism, to start your body burning fat rather than the carbohydrates, stabilize your blood sugar levels, and break addictions.

During the first two weeks you must eat no more than 20 grams of carbohydrate per day, the majority of which should come from vegetables and salads. You have to cut all breads, pasta, coffee, and alcohol, to mention but a few, from your diet. You may experience headaches, and other typical detoxification feelings during these weeks, but ultimately it is well worth while.
Foods allowed during first two week induction phase include:
- Fish, including: tuna, salmon, sole, trout
- Fowl, including: chicken, turkey, duck, goose
- Shellfish, including: lobster, squid, prawns
- Meats, including: pork, beef, lamb, bacon, ham
- Also: eggs, up to 90grams of most cheeses a day and 230-340 grams of salads.

On Going Weight Loss
The difference between Induction and the on going weight loss (OWL) phases of atkins is that you are allowed to consume more carbohydrates. You increase your carb intake up to 25 grams a day and continue to increase by 5 grams a week until you are no longer losing weight.

PreMaintenance
In this phase of the atkins diet you introduce more varied carbs slowly into you diet. You monitor how much carb you can eat without putting on weight.

Lifetime Maintenance
Following the pre maintenance phase you should know what you can eat to stick to you target weight.....

Body-Clock Diet

This diet is specifically aimed at women and in particular, women who find they are constantly yo-yo dieting. Working with the menstrual cycle you will tailor the diet to suit your own body clock. There are three slimming plan options to choose from depending on the level of weight loss required. The diet basics are a reduced fat, high carbohydrate eating plan but, unlike other diets, it is specifically designed to fit in with your menstrual cycle.

Split into 3 seperate phases, with the first phase started during your period followed by the other two phases until your next period when you repeat the sequence.

Phase A
For most women, this phase takes around 14 days and is the most calorie reduced phase.

Phase B
This phase starts when your mood begins to change. For most women this will be about 10-14 days before the period is due. The calorie content is increased slightly to allow for some sweet or starchy treats. Most women feel a more distinct change of mood a few days before their period, becoming a little more tense or even tearful and perhaps getting cravings. This is the time to switch to Phase C.

Phase C
This is usually confined to the last week of your cycle - often just a few days before the period when your mood is lowest and cravings worst. The calorie allowance is relatively generous in this phase allowing for 3 starchy or sugary treats including chocolate. The time spent on this phase should be kept to a minimum as it does have the higher calorie allowance. Even though you will still be loosing fat, you may still gain a little weight due to fluid retention.

The 3 options available for you on this diet are:-
Plan 1000 - A 1000 calorie a day option
Plan 1250 - A 1250 calorie a day option
Plan 1500 - A 1500 calorie a day option

Plan 1000 is intended for women with the least weight to lose and Plan 1500 is for those with most to lose. The reason for this is Plan 1500 will not trigger the 'famine response' in those with more weight to lose.

Body-Clock Diet Rules
The following basic rules apply whichever plan you are on.
- Each day choose one 'breakfast', one 'light meal' and one 'main meal'.
- In Phase C you are encouraged to have 3 snack/treats a day in addition to your set meals and should preferably be starchy carbohydrate foods to help prevent cravings.
- It is important to vary choices from day to day to get a wide variety of nutrients.
- Always keep to the choices in each particular phase. Do not 'mix' phases.
- Keep to the weights and measures shown.
- With meat, remove all visible fat before cooking and grill rather than fry.

Allowances

Milk - in addition to the meal choices you are allowed an extra 300ml skimmed OR 200ml semi-skimmed milk a day. You can also choose 2x125g diet yoghurt or 2x100g low-fat fromage frais.

Salad - in addition to the meal choices, eat a generous mixed vegetable salad each day (from the Ad Lib list) either with a meal or as a snack.

Fruit - Eat 100 calories worth of fruit a day selected from Healthy Extras 100 list.

Ad Libs

Have as much as you like from the following:-

- Unlimited amounts of water, diet soft drinks, unsugared tea, coffee or herbal tea.
- Virtually unlimited lettuce, tomato, cucumber, celery, cress, radish, bean sprouts, onions, garlic, cauliflower, courgettes, peppers, mushrooms, cabbage, carrot and spinach.
- Unlimited herbs and spices.
- Artificial sweeteners.

Healthy Xtras 100

Each item amounts to 100 calories. For example, you can have five satsumas for 100 calories.

Fruit:
- 1 medium banana
- 2 x 1/2 average size grapefruit
- 2 slices honeydew melon
- 2 medium apples, pears, oranges or peaches
- 5 satsumas
- 100g semi-dried apricots
- 1 x 250ml carton of long-life fruit juice

Starchy things:
- 1 standard shredded wheat plus 100ml skimmed milk
- 1 medium slice wholemeal bread plus 1/3 small banana mashed as spread
- 2 rye crisp breads spread with 1 tsp diet coleslaw
- 1 medium slice wholemeal bread, toasted, covered with 2 tsp baked beans
- 1 mini-pitta bread smeared with 15g houmous

Other:
- 150g natural low fat yoghurt with 1 tsp honey
- 2 x 100g low fat fromage frais fruit flavours
- 125g low fat yoghurt and rich tea biscuit

Wicked Treats 100

Each item amounts to 100 calories. For example, you can have one bag of peanuts for 100 calories.

Tea-time things:
- 2 x shortbread, ginger nut, rich tea or butter crunch biscuits
- 1 1/2 bourbons, chocolate chip cookies or custard creams
- 1 x 25g bag peanuts
- 1 medium slice wholemeal bread, low fat spread, smear of honey or jam

Chocolaty things:
- two-fifths of a 50g bar of plain, milk or white chocolate
- 1 chocolate digestive biscuit
- 2 chocolate-topped orange cake-biscuits

Alcohol:
- 1 x 150ml glass dry or medium white, red or rose wine

- 1 x 300ml ordinary strength lager, beer or cider
- 2 x 300ml low alcohol lager, beer or cider
- 2 singles or 1 double gin, whiskey, brandy, vodka, rum or tequila

Healthy Xtras 250
Each item amounts to 250 calories. For example, you can have twelve satsumas for 250 calories.
Fruit:
- 2 x large bananas
- 3 x small bananas
- 5 x medium apples, pears, oranges or peaches
- 12 x satsumas
Starchy things:
- 50g most breakfast cereals plus 150ml skimmed milk
- 1 wholemeal pitta bread, warmed, with 50g houmous and 6 stoned black olives
- 2 medium slices of wholemeal toast plus 150g baked beans

Wicked Treats 250
Each item amounts to 250 calories. For example, you can have 3 x 25g bags of peanuts for 250 calories.
Tea-time things:
- 5 x shortbread, ginger nut, rich tea or butter crunch biscuits
- 4 x bourbon, chocolate chip cookies or custard cream biscuits
- 3 x 25g bags of peanuts
- 1 x 75g jam doughnut
- 75g slice of cake
Chocolaty things:
- 1 only of any 50g plain, milk or white chocolate bar
- 1 1/2 flaky chocolate bars
- 2 milky-filled chocolate bars
- 2 large chocolate wafer biscuits
- 3 chocolate digestive biscuits
Alcohol:
- 2 x 150ml glass dry or medium white, red or rose wine
- 2 x 300ml ordinary strength lager, beer or cider
- 5 x 300ml low alcohol lager, beer or cider
- 4 singles or 2 doubles gin, whiskey, brandy, vodka, rum or tequila

Body-Clock Plan 1000
Averaging 1000 calories a day this is a short, sharp diet. Remember to select only the menu options from whichever phase of the plan you're currently going through. Never mix phases. Each day, select one breakfast, one light meal and one main meal.

Phase A Breakfasts
- 25g branflakes or standard shredded wheat, milk from allowance, fruit from allowance
- 1 medium slice wholemeal bread, toasted, smear of low fat spread and fruit from allowance
- 1 small banana mashed in 2 tsp of half cream
Phase A Light Meals
- 200g jacket baked potato, filled with 150g baked beans. Salad or fruit from allowance

- 2 x medium slices wholemeal bread smeared with low fat spread, 65g lean ham. Salad or fruit from allowance
- 1 hard boiled egg mashed with 1 tsp low fat mayonnaise, served on 1 medium wholemeal bap smeared with 2 tsp low fat sunflower spread. Salad or fruit from allowance.

Phase A Main Meals
- Turkey stir-fry. 1 piece of fruit from allowance
- Stuffed peppers. 50g piece Edam, Gouda or low fat soft cheese and a cracker or rye crispbread
- Vegetable Moussaka. 1 piece of fruit from allowance

Phase B Breakfasts
- Choose from Phase A selections
Phase B Light Meals
- Choose from Phase A selections
Phase B Main Meals
- Choose from Phase A selections
Phase B Snacks/Treats
- Choose an item from Healthy Xtras 100 list or Wicked Treats 100 list

Phase C Breakfasts
- Choose from Phase A selections
Phase C Light Meals
- Choose from Phase A selections
Phase C Main Meals
- Choose from Phase A selections
Phase C Snacks/Treats
- Choose three items from Healthy Xtras 100 list or Wicked Treats 100 list

Body-Clock Plan 1250
Averaging 1250 calories a day this is a medium term diet. Remember to select only the menu options from whichever phase of the plan you're currently going through. Never mix phases. Each day, select one breakfast, one light meal and one main meal.

Phase A Breakfasts
- 25g branflakes or standard shredded wheat, milk from allowance, fruit from allowance
- 1 medium slice wholemeal bread, toasted, smear of low fat spread and fruit from allowance
- 1 small banana mashed in 2 tsp of half cream
Phase A Light Meals
- 200g jacket baked potato, filled with 150g baked beans. Salad or fruit from allowance
- 2 x medium slices wholemeal bread smeared with low fat spread, 65g lean ham. Salad or fruit from allowance
- 1 hard boiled egg mashed with 1 tsp low fat mayonnaise, served on 1 medium wholemeal bap smeared with 2 tsp low fat sunflower spread. Salad or fruit from allowance
Phase A Main Meals
- Bacon and Potato Bake. Green salad from Ad Libs plus 62g frozen fruit mousse
- Spaghetti Bolognese. Green salad from Ad Libs. Fresh fruit and/or low fat yoghurt from allowances
- Eggs Florentine. 75g new potatoes. Fresh fruit or low fat yoghurt from allowance

Phase B Breakfasts
- 1/2 grapefruit. 1 medium slice wholemeal toast with thin smear of low fat spread
- 1boiled/poached egg. 1 medium slice wholemeal toast with low fat spread
- 1 shredded wheat. 150ml skimmed milk. 1/2 medium sized banana chopped in

Phase B Light Meals
- 200g jacket baked potato filled with 40g reduced fat cheddar. 1 orange/apple/pear
- 2 medium slices wholemeal bread, smear of low fat spread. 25g lean ham. 1 sliced tomato. 1 orange/apple
- 1 rye crispbread topped with 1 hard boiled egg finely diced with low fat mayonnaise. 1 orange/apple/pear

Phase B Main Meals
- Choose from Phase A selections

Phase B Snacks/Treats
- Choose three items from Healthy Xtras 100 list or Wicked Treats 100 list

Phase C Breakfasts
- Choose from Phase B selections

Phase C Light Meals
- Choose from Phase B selections

Phase C Main Meals
- Choose from Phase B selections

Phase C Snacks/Treats
- Choose two items from Healthy Xtras 250 list or two items from Wicked Treats 250 list PLUS one item from Healthy Xtras 100 list or Wicked Treats 100 list

Body-Clock Plan 1500
Averaging 1500 calories a day this is a longer term diet. Remember to select only the menu options from whichever phase of the plan you're currently going through. Never mix phases. Each day, select one breakfast, one light meal and one main meal.

Phase A Breakfasts
- 1/2 grapefruit. 1 medium slice wholemeal toast with thin smear of low fat spread
- 1boiled/poached egg. 1 medium slice wholemeal toast with low fat spread
- 1 shredded wheat. 150ml skimmed milk. 1/2 medium sized banana chopped in

Phase A Light Meals
- 200g jacket baked potato filled with 40g reduced fat cheddar. 1 orange/apple/pear
- 2 medium slices wholemeal bread, smear of low fat spread. 25g lean ham. 1 sliced tomato. 1 orange/apple
- 1 rye crispbread topped with 1 hard boiled egg finely diced with low fat mayonnaise. 1 orange/apple/pear

Phase A Main Meals
- Tuna and egg salad. Summer pudding
- Turkey two-pepper salad. Strawberry parfait
- Gammon and spicy pineapple. Potatoes and vegetables. 100g low fat fromage frais

Phase B Breakfasts
- Choose from Phase A selections

Phase B Light Meals

- Choose from Phase A selections
Phase B Main Meals
- Choose from Phase A selections
Phase B Snacks/Treats
- Choose an item from Healthy Xtras 250 list or Wicked Treats 250 list

Phase C Breakfasts
- Choose from Phase A selections
Phase C Light Meals
- Choose from Phase A selections
Phase C Main Meals
- Choose from Phase A selections
Phase C Snacks/Treats
- Choose three items from Healthy Xtras 250 list or Wicked Treats 250 list

Body-Clock Diet Recipes

Turkey Stir-Fry
Serves 4;   350 calories per serving

2 spring onions, sliced
2 cloves garlic, crushed
2.5cm piece root ginger, grated
1 stick celery, thinly sliced
1 medium sized onion, diced
350g turkey breast, sliced and chopped
1 green pepper, de-seeded and diced
100g baby sweetcorn
100g frozen peas or broccoli florets
2 tsp soy sauce
1 tsp sherry
1 tsp chilli sauce
1 pinch Chinese 5-spice
4 tsp stock
1 tsp lemon juice
225g instant egg noodles
tsp corn or sunflower oil

Heat the oil in a wok or large frying pan. Gently fry the spring onions, garlic and ginger until soft. Add the celery, onion and turkey. Stir-fry over a high heat for about 3 minutes. Add the remaining vegetables and stir for another 3 minutes. Mix the soy sauce, sherry, chilli sauce, spice, stock and lemon juice and stir into the wok. Bring to the boil. Cook the egg noodles in lightly salted water, and serve with the stir-fry.

Stuffed Peppers
Serves 4;   200 calories per serving

100g brown rice

4 green or red peppers
1 medium onion, finely chopped
40g sunflower seeds
40g dried apricots
1/2 tsp dried thyme or 1 tsp fresh thyme
1 size 3 egg
250ml tomato juice
salt

Simmer the rice n lightly boiling water for 20 minutes. Drain. Halve the peppers and de-seed. Mix the onion, sunflower seeds, apricots, thyme and egg with the rice, and stuff the mixture into the peppers. Place, with tomato juice, in a hot oven and bake for 30-40 minutes.

Vegetable Moussaka
Serves 4;   350 calories per serving

2 medium sized aubergines
225g sliced mushrooms
2 cloves crushed garlic
4 sticks of sliced celery
2 medium sliced leeks
2 x 400g cans chopped tomatoes
450ml semi-skimmed milk
3 heaped tsp flour
100g low fat soft cheese
50g half fat grated cheddar
1 tsp sunflower oil
2 tsp salt

Cut the aubergines into 1cm slices. Sprinkle with the salt and leave for 30 minutes to absorb the bitter juices. Rinse off the salt with cold water and dab dry. Heat the oil in a pan and gently fry the mushrooms and garlic for 3 minutes. Blanch the celery and leeks in boiling water for 2 minutes and drain. Drain the tomatoes. Mix 4 tsp of the milk with the flour to make a smooth paste. Stir in the remaining milk and heat gently in a saucepan until it thickens. Blend in the soft cheese. Spread out half the aubergine slices to cover the base of a large ovenproof dish. Add the mushrooms and garlic mixture, spreading it out. Add half the tomatoes to make another layer. Then a layer of the leeks and celery. Then the rest of the aubergines, and the rest of the tomatoes. Top with the sauce, sprinkled with the grated cheese. Bake in a pre-heated moderate oven 200C/400F/Gas 6 until brown (25-30 minutes). Serve with lettuce and black olive salad.

Bacon and Potato Bake
Serves 4;   380 calories per serving

675g peeled potatoes
1 egg size 3
50g low fat spread
225g lean back bacon
200g can sweetcorn, drained

225g cottage cheese with chives
salt and pepper to taste
chopped fresh chives, to garnish

Boil the potatoes until soft, and drain off the water. Beat the egg in a cup and add to the potatoes with the low fat spread. Mash with a fork until creamy. Grill the bacon and cut or break into small pieces. Stir the sweetcorn and cottage cheese into the mash, mixing thoroughly. Add salt and pepper to taste. Spread the mixture into a large ovenproof dish. Place in a pre-heated hot oven 220C/425F/Gas 7 and bake until it begins to brown (25-30 minutes). Sprinkle with chopped chives and serve with a green salad.

Spaghetti Bolognese
Serves 4;   450 calories per serving

2 medium onions, finely chopped
3 cloves garlic, sliced
2 sticks celery, sliced
2 medium carrots, grated
450g lean minced beef
400g can tomatoes
2 tsp tomato puree
pinch dried oregano
200g spaghetti
black pepper to taste
1 tsp olive or sunflower oil

Heat the oil in a pan and gently fry the onions, garlic and celery until softened. Add the carrots and mince and stir-cook until the mince is brown. Add the tomatoes, tomato puree and oregano. Bring to the boil, cover and simmer for 30 minutes. Meanwhile, cook the spaghetti in boiling lightly salted water for 10-12 minutes. Drain and serve topped with the Bolognese sauce. season with black pepper to taste.

Eggs Florentine
Serves 4;   400 calories per serving

8 size 3 eggs
675 frozen spinach
black pepper
large pinch of ground nutmeg
50g low fat spread
2 heaped tsp plain flour
450ml skimmed milk
100g reduced fat hard cheese, grated

Hard boil the eggs. Meanwhile, steam the spinach and thoroughly drain it. Season with pepper and nutmeg and place in an ovenproof dish. Slice the eggs and arrange on top of the spinach. Mix the low fat spread, flour and skimmed milk in a pan, bring to the boil and whisk until thickened. Stir in the grated cheese and pour over the eggs. Grill until cheese sauce bubbles.

Body For Life

Imagine, just 12 weeks from now, having the lean, healthy body you've always wanted and *not* having to turn your life upside down to get it. Don't just imagine it -- make it a reality! Bill Phillips is here with his best-selling Body-for-LIFE weight loss plan and his brand-new Body-for-LIFE Success Journal, which guides you through the plan day by day and makes it easier than ever to reach your goals. It's like having Bill Phillips there with you, every step of the way!

Start the Body-*for*-LIFE program today:
- **Maximize your results**: Identify your twelve-week goals
- **Get ready for Day 1**: Make a plan you can stick to
- **Blast fat and build muscle**: Start the super efficient workout plan
- **Fire up your metabolism**: Try the simple, satisfying eating plan and find out which foods are best for you. Plus, check out a sample day's menu.

This journal entry involves three exercises. In the first exercise, you will write down five specific 12-week goals. If you want to gain muscle and lose fat, you might write the following goals:
- "Within 12 weeks, I will gain five pounds of muscle!"
- "Within 12 weeks, I will lose 20 pounds of fat!"

By composing sentences like these, by defining and stating your wish and by setting a deadline (within 12 weeks), you'll be transforming your dreams into goals. Once you clarify your goals, be sure to read them first thing in the morning and again at night.

In the next exercise, identify your reasons for achieving your 12-week goals. What I've discovered is that the more clear you are about why those goals are important to you, the more likely it is you'll succeed. It's not complicated at all to identify reasons for making changes to improve your health and fitness. There are countless reasons for wanting to become healthier, stronger and more energetic. Be sure to write down three that have meaning to you. And please read your reasons every time you review your goals.

The next exercise is called Transforming Patterns of Action. To complete this exercise, you identify three habits you have now, which you'll need to transform in order for you to move forward and become a success. For example, if one of your goals is to lose 20 pounds of fat within 12 weeks, it's very likely you will need to begin carefully planning nutritious meals, instead of just eating carelessly. I've discovered the best way to develop new, healthy habits is to identify ones that are not working for you and pretty much do the opposite.

By clearly stating your goals, by identifying reasons why those goals are important to you and by writing down three old, "unauthorized" patterns of action and three new, effective ones, you're crossing the abyss between knowing what to do and actually doing it.

This journal entry involves three exercises. The first one is called the Power Mindset. This exercise helps you focus on and prioritize your daily Body-*for*-LIFE activities. You see, in order to experience an extraordinary transformation in just 12 weeks, you need to make progress every day. And by simply deciding what five things you can do tomorrow to move forward in the direction of your 12-week goals, you will stay on course and remain focused.

Next is the Universal Law of Reciprocation exercise. In order to make the successful transformation you've decided to make, you will need support and encouragement: And the best way to receive is to give. This simple exercise creates immediate results that will increase your energy and confidence. When you say something as simple as, "I appreciate your support!" or, "Good work!" you not only give someone else a boost, but according to the Universal Law of Reciprocation, you will receive more positive energy than you give.

Both of these exercises should be planned during your evening journaling session. During the course of the next day, or your next evening journaling session, review what you planned to do, and if you followed your plan, write "Success!" in the Actual column. If you did not achieve your daily goal, write "Setback," and be sure to try harder tomorrow.

The next mindset exercise is Focus on Progress, Not Perfection. You should complete this exercise only during your evening journaling session. What you'll do here is reflect on your day and write down three things you did very well that helped you move forward. This exercise gives you positive reinforcement and helps you build momentum, because you're giving yourself credit where credit is due. When you look for three things you've done right that day, you'll find them! Your final assignment is to identify just one thing you can do even better tomorrow than you did today.

How to Train

- Weight train, intensely, for no more than 46 minutes, three times per week: Monday, Wednesday, and Friday. Perform 20 minutes of aerobic exercise, first thing in the morning on an empty stomach, three times per week: Tuesday, Thursday, and Saturday. Take Sunday off -- it's your free day.

- Alternate training the major muscles of the upper and lower body. For example, the first week, train upper body on Monday, lower body on Wednesday, and upper body on Friday. The second week, train lower body on Monday, upper body on Wednesday, and lower body on Friday.

- Perform two exercises for each major muscle group of the upper body, which includes: chest, shoulders, back, triceps, and biceps; and for the lower body: quadriceps, hamstrings, and calves. Train the abdominal muscles after lower body.

- Select one exercise for each muscle group and conduct five sets, starting with a set of 12 reps, then increasing the weight and doing 10 reps, adding more weight and doing eight reps, adding more weight for six reps. Then reduce the weight, do 12 more reps, and immediately go to another set of 12 reps of another exercise for that muscle group.

- On all lifts, use a cadence of two seconds (say "I am building my Body-*for*-LIFE") to lower the weight and one second (say "Body-*for*-LIFE") to lift it, and "hold" in the top and bottom positions for a count of "one."

- For each muscle group, rest for one minute between the first four sets. Then complete the final two sets with no rest in between. Wait two minutes before moving on to your next muscle group. Complete this pattern five times for the upper body training experience and four times for the lower body training experience.

Nutrition Rules to Remember

- Eat six small meals a day, one every two to three hours.
- Eat a portion of protein and carbohydrates with each meal.
- Add a portion of vegetables to at least two meals daily.
- A portion is the amount of an authorized food approximately the size of the palm of your hand or your clenched fist.
- Consume one tablespoon of unsaturated oil daily or three portions of salmon per week.
- Drink at least 10 cups of water a day.
- Use performance-nutrition shakes if necessary to make sure you're consuming optimal levels of required nutrients.
- Plan your meals in advance, and record what you eat.
- Plan your grocery list.
- Once a week, on your free day, eat whatever you want.

Basic Eating Plan

Choose a portion of protein and carbohydrates from each section to make a meal. Add a serving of vegetable to at least two of your daily meals.

Proteins
- Chicken breast, turkey breast, lean ground turkey, swordfish, orange roughy, haddock, salmon, tuna, crab, lobster, shrimp, top round steak, top sirloin steak, lean ground beef, buffalo, lean ham, egg whites or substitutes, low-fat cottage cheese

Carbs
- Baked potato, sweet potato, yam, squash, pumpkin, steamed brown rice, steamed wild rice, pasta, oatmeal, barley, beans, corn, strawberries, melon, apple, orange, fat-free yogurt, whole-wheat bread

Vegetables
- Broccoli, asparagus, lettuce, carrots, cauliflower, green beans, green peppers, mushroom, spinach, tomato, peas, brussels sprouts, artichoke, cabbage, celery, zucchini, cucumber, onion

A Day on Body-for-Life

Breakfast: Zesty Breakfast Burrito
Fill a small whole-wheat tortilla with four scrambled egg whites or Egg Beaters. Add one tablespoon of salsa, half a tablespoon of low-fat shredded cheddar cheese, and one tablespoon of low-fat sour cream. Roll and serve along with a tall glass of ice water.

Midmorning: Chocolate-Mint Nutrition Shake
Mix one serving of a chocolate Myoplex according to directions. Then add three drops of peppermint extract and three ice cubes. Blend at high speed for 45 seconds and serve.

Lunch: Grilled Chicken Soup
In a small sauce pan, mix one can of chicken broth; a sliced, grilled chicken breast; a portion of cooked barley; and a handful of your favourite mixed vegetables. (The frozen ones are not only convenient, they're just as nutritious as fresh vegetables.) Warm over medium heat for five minutes

and serve with two cups of ice water or iced tea.

Midafternoon: Strawberry-Frost Nutrition Shake

Mix one serving of strawberry Myoplex according to directions. Add three ice cubes. Blend at high speed for 45 seconds and serve.

Dinner: Grilled Salmon and Potato

Prepare a salmon steak by squeezing fresh lemon juice over it. Grill salmon for 10 to 15 minutes or until it flakes easily when tested with a fork. Serve with a baked potato, steamed spinach, and ice water.

Late Evening: Cinnamon Roll Supreme Nutrition Shake

Mix one serving of a vanilla Myoplex powder according to directions. Then add one half teaspoon ground cinnamon, one teaspoon fat-free Butter Buds, and three ice cubes. Blend at high speed for 45 seconds and serve.

Example 7 Day Diet & Exercise Routine

Monday

Meal 1: Myoplex Lite shake
Meal 2: Lean sausage, 1 cup Cream of Wheat
Meal 3: Chicken breast, 3/4 cup brown rice, salsa, salad
Meal 4: Fajitas: chicken breast cut in strips, whole-wheat tortilla, salsa, fat free cheese
Meal 5: 1 cup low-fat cottage cheese, 1 apple
Meal 6: Egg salad (5 boiled egg whites, fat free mayo) on whole wheat bread
Workout: Interval training on elliptical machine; 20 minutes

Tuesday

Meal 1: Shake (protein powder and banana blended with ice) and a salad
Meal 2: A green bell pepper stuffed with lean ground beef, 3/4 cup brown rice and onion
Meal 3: Myoplex Lite shake
Meal 4: Fried rice (4 egg whites/1 whole egg, 3/4 cup brown rice, onion, bell pepper and salsa)
Meal 5: 1 cup low-fat cottage cheese on a baked potato, topped with salsa
Meal 6: Myoplex Lite shake
Workout: Upper body workout with weights (back, biceps, triceps, shoulders, chest); 40 minutes

Wednesday

Meal 1:1 egg-white omelette (4 eggs), 1/2 cup oatmeal
Meal 2:Lean sausage, 1 cup Cream of Wheat
Meal 3:Myoplex Lite shake
Meal 4:Lean hamburger patty on whole wheat bread with lettuce, onion and tomato
Meal 5:Shake (protein powder and banana blended with ice)
Meal 6:1 cup low-fat cottage cheese, 8 ounces sugar free/fat free yogurt
Workout: Interval training on elliptical machine; 20 minutes

Thursday

Meal 1: 1 cup low-fat cottage cheese, 1 apple
Meal 2: Egg salad (5 boiled egg whites, fat free mayo) on whole wheat bread
Meal 3: Chicken breast, 3/4 cup brown rice, salsa, salad
Meal 4: Fajitas (chicken breast cut in strips, whole-wheat tortilla, salsa, fat free cheese)
Meal 5: Myoplex Lite shake
Meal 6: Lean sausage, 1 cup Cream of Wheat
Workout: Lower body workout with weights (abs, hamstrings, quads, calves); 40 minutes

Friday

Meal 1: Shake (protein powder and banana blended with ice) and a salad
Meal 2: Fried rice (4 egg whites/1 whole egg, 3/4 cup brown rice, onion, bell pepper and salsa)
Meal 3: Myoplex Lite shake
Meal 4: A green bell pepper stuffed with lean ground beef, 3/4 cup brown rice and onion
Meal 5: 1 cup low-fat cottage cheese on a baked potato, topped with salsa
Meal 6: Myoplex Lite shake
Workout: Interval training on elliptical; 20 minutes

Saturday
Meal 1: 1 egg-white omelette (4 eggs), 1/2 cup oatmeal
Meal 2: Lean sausage, 1 cup Cream of Wheat
Meal 3: Myoplex Lite shake
Meal 4: Lean hamburger patty on whole wheat bread with lettuce, onion and tomato
Meal 5: Shake (protein powder and banana blended with ice)
Meal 6: 1 cup low-fat cottage cheese, 8 ounces sugar free/fat free yogurt
Workout: Day off

Sunday
Breakfast: Donuts
Lunch: Chinese buffet
Dinner: Bacon cheeseburger, tator tots, large grape slush
Snacks: A large cappuccino and Oreos
Workout: Upper body workout with weights (back, biceps, triceps, shoulders, chest), 40 minutes

Cabbage Soup Diet

The Soup Diet is based on a fat-burning soup that contains negligible calories. The more soup you eat the more weight you should lose. It allows people to eat as much Cabbage Soup as they want each day, which should sound appealing to dieters. After all, dieters love to hear that they can eat unlimited amounts of food and still lose weight fast.

The Diet relies on eating strange and bizarre combinations of food that nearly force you to starve each day. Dieters are allowed all the water and cabbage soup they want, plus a very restricted set of other foods.

A running myth suggests that this diet originated at any number of hospitals, but thus far, no medical facilities have claimed it as their own. Consensus is that the diet is effective for temporarily losing a few pounds. However, this is not a very nutritionally sound plan and certainly not one to live on.

The 7 Days Diet Plan

Eat as much soup as you desire for seven days and you can lose 10 to 15 pounds. The recipe varies slightly, but includes a variety of low-calorie vegetables such as cabbage, onions, and tomatoes, flavoured with bouillon, onion soup mix, and tomato juice. Each day of the seven-day program has specific foods that must be eaten, including potatoes, fruit juice, many vegetables, and on one day, beef.

Day One:
Eat only fruit, all the fruit you want except banana.
Drink unsweetened tea, black coffee, cranberry juice, and water.
Eat as much soup as you like.

Day Two:
All you want - fresh, raw, or cooked vegetables of your choice. Stay away from dry beans, peas, and sweet corn. Reward yourself with a big baked potato with butter for dinner. Eat as much soup as you like but no fruit for today.

Day Three:
Combine days one and two, eat as much fruit, vegetables, and soup, as you like but no baked potato.

Day Four:
Eat as many as eight bananas and drink as many glasses of skim milk as you would like on this day, along with your soup. This day is supposed to lessen your desire for sweets.

Day Five:
You may have 10-20 ounces of beef (300-500g) and a large tin or up to six fresh tomatoes. Drink at least 6 to 8 glasses of water this day to wash the uric acid from your body. Eat your soup at least once today. You may eat broiled or baked chicken (skinless) instead of beef. If you prefer, you can substitute broiled fish for the beef.

Day Six:

Eat beef and vegetables today. You can even have two or three steaks if you like, with fresh vegetables or salad. NO BAKED POTATO. Eat your soup at least once.

Day Seven:

Eat all you want of brown rice, unsweetened fruit juices, and vegetables. Be sure to eat your soup at least once to day. No bread, alcohol, or carbonated beverages, not even diet soda.

The Curves Fitness Program

The Curves fitness program is an efficient 30-minute exercise routine that is advertised as being "Fast, Effective, and Fun." It combines cardiovascular training with strength training of both the upper and lower body.

The basic workout consists of the following:
1. Warm-up
2. Twenty minutes of aerobic movement at a sustained target heart rate
3. Three sets of strength training on all major muscle groups
4. Cool down
5. Stretching routine

The program is called the Quickfit system and uses a "circuit" that consists of a series of exercise machines and recovery stations. The machines are hydraulic-based, meaning a participant uses her own strength to work against the machine. These machines enable the individual to work two muscle groups at a time, while conventional machines work on only one muscle.

The circuit consists of eight or 12 different machines usually arranged in a circle. You can join the circuit at any time as long as there is a vacant spot. The machines emphasize exercising various areas of the body. For example, machines include a biceps arm curl, a chest pull, an adductor/abductor for the thighs, and a "squat" for the gluteus maximus. The participant completes as many repetitions on the machines as she can in 30 seconds.

The circuit also alternates with "recovery stations" that are placed between the machines. These are simply wooden step-down boards. You can do just about anything-shake, jog, stretch, or dance-on the recovery stations as long as you keep moving. The recovery enables you to keep up a target heart rate while resting your muscles. During the 30-minute program, the circuit is completed three times, moving from machine to recovery station and then to the next machine. There are also breaks to check your target heart rate and adjust your workout if necessary.

The program recommends starting to "cool down" for approximately three minutes before leaving the circuit by reducing the aerobic intensity of your movement. The circuit training is then followed by three minutes of 12 simple stretches to prevent muscle injury and provide flexibility. There are charts with pictures of each stretch that demonstrate exactly what to do. Stretching is important, especially for women over the age of 50 and those with joint, back, or autoimmune issues.

Women who have previously found it difficult to keep up an exercise regimen like the fact that they do not have to adjust each machine or change weight stacks, which can be time-consuming and frustrating. Also, the circuit is automatic, so participants do not have to plan out each step. The drawback to this is that it does not provide an individualized program, although the pace can be adjusted. The intensity of this workout may fall short of what some women desire.

The program also has its limitations. Many facilities are cramped and crowded with machines that are positioned too close together and are well-worn. There are limited hours, especially on weekends, and there is no provision for baby-sitting.

The Curves Diet Plan

The Curves diet has been a topic of conversation and controversy among health professionals and dieticians. This plan is exclusive to the Curves franchise and consists of two separate diet strategies: one is a Low-Carbohydrate Plan, which is not as stringent as the Atkins Diet Plan; the other is a Low-Calorie Plan, which also stresses lowering simple carbohydrates in the daily diet. Nutrition professionals cannot promote any other plans on the premises. However, members are free to discuss any diet plan they like and exchange recipes and advice while on the circuit.

It has been found that in most Curves Centres, these particular diets are not excessively promoted. However, the plan does focus on diet cycling, carbohydrate intolerance, and calorie sensitivity. A more controversial piece of the package is the chain's promotion of its own line of dietary supplements, which includes its own brand of weight-loss shakes.

The Curves Weight-Loss and Fitness Programme

The Curves Weight-Loss and Fitness Programme has three components, each of which works in synergy with the others to help slim and tone your body while resetting your metabolism.

The Curves Meal Plan

The Curves Meal Plan reprogrammes your metabolism to work for you, not against you. It is designed to correct the disastrous effects of years of low-fat, low-calorie starvation diets and yo-yo dieting. You will choose between two different meal plans, each designed to accommodate different metabolic needs. The first meal plan, the Carbohydrate- Sensitive Plan, is a high-protein, low-carbohydrate meal plan for those of you who are carbohydrate-intolerant. The second, the Calorie- Sensitive Plan, is designed for those of you who are not good candidates for the advantages of a high-protein meal plan. I will explain the difference between these two plans in Chapters 2 and 3. In Chapter 3, I have also provided a short quiz that will help you determine which meal plan you should follow. Both meal plans are divided into three phases.

PHASE 1   GET OFF TO A GREAT START. The first phase is the strictest phase of the programme. It jump-starts your weight loss by shifting your body into fat-burning mode. Most women lose 6 to 10 pounds fairly quickly. Phase 1 is the most restrictive part of the diet, but you are only on it for one or two weeks, depending on how much weight you need to lose.

PHASE 2   REACH YOUR GOAL . In Phase 2, you are eating considerably more food but still losing weight (about one to two pounds per week). You stay on Phase 2 until you reach your desired weight, hit a plateau, or need a break from dieting.

PHASE 3   RETRAIN YOUR METABOLISM. Phase 3 is the fulfilment of the Curves Promise: permanent weight loss without permanent dieting. In Phase 3, you are no longer on a diet. On most days, you will be eating between 2,500 and 3,000 calories, yet you will keep the weight off. You will learn how and why this is possible in Chapter 2, Metabolic Magic: Escaping the Diet Trap of Slow Metabolism.

I understand how busy women are today, so my goal is to make this programme as easy to follow as possible. In Chapters 5 and 6, you will find seven weeks of Curves Meal Plan sample menus, so you'll never run out of ideas about what to eat. In the Curves Daily Planner I also provide weekly shopping lists, recipes and charts to help you plan your meals and track your progress. I promise, following this Curves Meal Plan is not going to be a chore. And don't worry, you won't even have to prepare different meals for your family. As you will see, it's easy to stay on your meal plan and still satisfy your family without a lot of extra work.

The Curves Workout

The Curves At-Home Workout will help build new calorie-burning muscle while you slim down and tone up. The 30-minute regimen is a combination of strength training, aerobics and stretching. I show you how to do a complete upper- and lower-body workout while exercising your cardiovascular system at the same time. The workout is efficient, effective and enjoyable. The only equipment you need is a simple, inexpensive exercise resistance tube you can buy at any sporting-goods store, or even on the Internet. The best news is that you only need to do these exercises three times a week to achieve spectacular results. My programme is designed to accommodate the needs of women regardless of their level of fitness. It enables you to go at your own pace.

The Curves Supplement Regimen

Most of us do not get all the nutrients we need from food alone. Modern food-processing techniques have stripped the vitamins, minerals and other beneficial chemicals out of the food supply, while adding tons of preservatives, insecticides, food dyes and other chemicals that are foreign to our bodies. Nutrient deficiency can sabotage your weight loss efforts by promoting food cravings and making you feel tired. In Chapter 11, I provide information on nutritional supplements that can help ensure that you are getting the nutrients your body needs. This is important, because even careful eaters may be nutrient deficient, and those you of who are not so careful are particularly at risk.

Eat Right For Your Type

According to Dr. Peter DÁdamo, author of Eat Right For Your Type, a chemical reaction occurs between your blood and the foods you eat. This reaction is part of your genetic inheritance. This reaction is caused by a factor called Lectins. Lectins, abundant and diverse proteins found in foods, have agglutinating properties that affect your blood. So when you eat a food containing protein lectins that are incompatible with your blood type antigen, the lectins target an organ or bodily system and begin to agglutinate blood cells in that area. Different lectins target different organs and body system.

Fortunately, most lectins found in the diet are not quite so life threatening, although they can cause a variety of other problems, especially if they are specific to a particular blood type. For the most part your immune systems protect you from lectins. Ninety-five percent of the lectins you absorb from your typical diets are sloughed off by the body. But at least five percent of the lectins you eat are filtered into the bloodstream and different reactions in different organs.

Your blood type diet is the restoration of your natural genetic rhythm. Your blood type diet works because you are able to follow a clear, logical, scientifically researched plan based on your cellular profile. Each food groups are divided into three categories: Highly beneficial (food that acts like Medicine), Foods allowed (food that are no harm to the blood type) and Foods not allowed (food that acts like a Poison)

Below is a summary of the various Blood Type Diet and detail plan of each one according to Dr. DÁdamo.

Blood Type Diet - Type O

Type Os thrive on intense physical exercise and animal protein. Unlike the other blood types, Type Os muscle tissue should be slightly on the acid side. Type Os can efficiently digest and metabolize meat because they tend to have high stomach-acid content. The success of the Type O Diet depends on the use of lean, chemical-free meats, poultry, and fish. Type Os don't find dairy products and grains quite as user friendly as do most of the other blood types.

The initial weight loss on the Type O Diet is by restricting consumption of grains, breads, legumes, and beans. The leading factor in weight gain for Type Os is the gluten found in wheat germ and whole wheat products, which interferes with insulin efficiency and slow down metabolic rate. Another factor that contribute to weight gain is certain beans and legumes (lentils and kidney beans) contain lectins that deposit in the muscle tissues making them less "charged" for physical activity. The third factor in Type O weight gain is that Type Os have a tendency to have low levels of thyroid hormone or unstable thyroid functions, which also cause metabolic problems. Therefore it is good to avoid food that inhibits thyroid hormone (cabbage, brussels sprouts, cauliflower, mustard green) but increase hormone production (kelp, seafood, iodized salt).

Several classes of vegetables can cause big problems for Type Os, such as the Brassica family (cabbage, cauliflower, etc.) can inhibit the thyroid function. Eat more vegetables that are high in Vitamin K, which helps the clotting factor which is weak in Type Os. The nightshade vegetables can cause lectin deposit in the tissue surrounding the joints.

Because of the high acidity stomach, Type Os should eat fruits of alkaline nature such as berries and plums..

Type Os should severely restrict the use of dairy products. Their system is not designed for the proper metabolism. If you are a Type O of African ancestry, you should eliminate dairy foods and eggs altogether.

Diet Profile:
High Protein: Meat eaters
Allowed:
Meat, fish, vegetables, fruit
Limited:
grains, beans, legumes
Food to avoid for Weight Loss purpose:
wheat, corn, kidney beans, navy beans, lentils, cabbage, Brussels sprouts, cauliflower, mustard greens
Food that help with Weight Loss:
kelp, seafood, salt, liver, red meat, kale, spinach, broccoli

Blood Type Diet - Type A

Type As flourish on vegetarian diets. Type As are predisposed to heart disease, cancer, and diabetes. It is particularly important for sensitive Type As to get their foods in as natural a state as possible: fresh, pure, and organic. When you get on the Type A Diet, you will naturally be thinner. If you are accustomed to eating meat, you'll lose weight rather rapidly in the beginning as you eliminate the toxic foods from your diet. And when you follow the Type diet, you can supercharge your immune system and potentially short-circuit the development of life-threatening diseases.

When Type As eat meat, they experience sluggishness. Type As have low stomach-acid content, therefore they have a hard time digesting meat. Since Type As eat very little animal protein, nuts and seeds supply an important protein component. Type As also thrive on the vegetable proteins found in beans and legumes, except those mentioned for the "Avoid" list. These beans can cause a decrease in insulin production, which may cause obesity and diabetes. Tofu should be a staple in the Type A Diet.

Dairy foods are also poorly digested by Type As, and can cause metabolic slowdown. Type As can tolerate small amounts of fermented dairy products such as yogurt, kefir, nonfat sour cream, and cultured dairy products.

Vegetables are vital to the Type A Diet, providing minerals, enzymes and antioxidants. Type A are very sensitive to the lectins in potatoes, sweet potatoes, yams, cabbage, tomatoes and peppers. They aggravate the delicate stomach of Type A. Type A should eat more fruits that are alkaline, avoid mangoes, papaya and oranges for they are not good for your digestive tract.

Diet Profile:
Vegetarian
Allowed:
vegetables, tofu, seafood, grains, beans, legumes, fruit

Food to avoid for Weight Loss purpose:
meat, dairy, kidney beans, lima beans, wheat
Food that help with Weight Loss:
vegetable oil, soy foods, vegetables, pineapple

Blood Type Diet - Type B

The sturdy and alert Type Bs are usually able to resist many of the most severe diseases common to modern life, such as heart disease and cancer. In fact, a Type B who carefully follows the recommended diet can often bypass severe disease and live a long and healthy life. Type Bs are more prone to immune-system disorders such as multiple sclerosis, lupus, and chronic fatigue syndrome.

The Type B Diet is balance and wholesome, including a wide variety of foods.

For Type Bs, the biggest factors in weight gain are corn, buckwheat, lentils, peanuts and sesame seeds. These foods have different lectin that affect the efficiency of the metabolic process, resulting in fatigue, fluid retention, and hypoglycemia. The gluten lectin in wheat germ and whole wheat products also adds to the problems cause by other metabolism-slowing foods.

It is important to leave off chicken for Type Bs. Chicken contains a Blood Type B agglutinating lectin in its muscle tissue, which attack the bloodstream and potentially lead to strokes and immune disorders. Type Bs thrive on deep-ocean fish, but should avoid all shellfish. The shellfish contain lectins that are disruptive to the Type B system.

Type B is the only blood type that can fully enjoy a variety of dairy foods. Most nuts and seeds (especially peanuts, sesame seeds and sunflower seeds) are not advised for Type Bs., they contain lectins that interfere with Type B insulin production.

Wheat is not tolerated well by most Type Bs. They contain a lectin that reduce insulin efficiency and failure to stimulate fat "burning". Rye contains a lectin that settles in the vascular system, causing blood disorders and potentially strokes. Corn and buckwheat are major factors in Type B weight gain, they contribute to a sluggish metabolism, insulin irregularity, fluid retention, and fatigue.

Eliminate tomatoes completely from Type B diet. It has lectins that irritate the stomach lining. Fruits and vegetables are generally well tolerated and should be taken generously.

Diet Profile:
Balanced omnivore
Allowed:
meat (no chicken), dairy, grains, beans, legumes, vegetables, fruit
Food to avoid for Weight Loss purpose:
corn, lentil, peanuts, sesame, seeds, buckwheat, wheat
Food that help with Weight Loss:
greens, eggs, venison, liver, liquorice, tea

Blood Type Diet - Type AB

Multiple antigens make Type ABs sometimes A-like with weak stomach acid, and sometimes B-like with genetically programmed for the consumption of meats. Type AB do best when their muscle tissues are slightly alkaline. Type ABs can't metabolize meat efficiently because of low stomach acid, so it is important to watch the portion size and frequency. Chicken has lectin that irritates the blood and digestive tracts of Type ABs also. Tofu is a good protein supplements for Type ABs. Nuts, seeds, beans and legumes present a mixed picture for Type ABs. Eat nuts and seeds in small amounts and with caution.

Type ABs can tolerate dairy foods fairly well. But watch out for excessive mucus production.

Generally Type ABs do well on grains, even wheat, but keep in mind that the inner kernel of the wheat grain is highly acid forming in the muscle for Type ABs. Type AB benefits from a diet rich in rice rather than pasta.

Type ABs has a weaker immune system, so you will benefit from the vegetables, which are high in phytocheicals and the more alkaline fruits, which can help to balance the grains that are acid forming in the muscle tissues. Tomatoes do not impose any ill effects on Type ABs.

Type AB should begin each day by drinking a glass of warm water with the freshly squeezed juice of half a lemon to cleanse the system of mucus accumulated while sleeping.

Diet Profile:
Mixed diet in moderation
Allowed:
meat, seafood, dairy, tofu, beans, legumes, grains, vegetables, fruits
Food to avoid for Weight Loss purpose:
red meat, kidney beans, lima beans, seeds, corn, buckwheat
Food that help with Weight Loss:
tofu, seafood, dairy, greens, kelp, pineapple

F-Plan Diet

This diet book by Audrey Eyton, originally published in 1982, was the first high-fibre diet, and remains the most famous of them all. The Complete F-Plan Diet was published a few years later. The theory behind this diet is that a high intake of dietary fibre (aka 'non-starch polysaccharides') quickly fills you up while you are eating. And because you have to do a lot of chewing, you each satiety point before you have eaten too many calories.

It offers bulk without calories (because fibre largely passes through the system undigested) and keeps hunger pangs at bay in between meals since high-fibre food takes longer to digest than low-fibre, refined foods.

F-Plan Diet and Health Issues

The F-Plan Diet is generally one of the healthiest to be found, even today. Although there is evidence that high intakes of wheat bran (found in the fibre-filler breakfast) can inhibit the absorption of minerals such as iron and calcium, a high-fibre diet is linked with less risk of some cancers. Recent research suggests that there is up to 40 percent less risk of bowel cancer with high fibre consumption.

The F-plan Diet may be low in essential fats from fish and plant oils depending on food choices made. Plenty of water or other low-calorie liquid should be taken on a high fibre diet.

Is the F-Plan Diet Scientifically Sound?

Most of the rationale for eating a high fibre diet while dieting is correct. However, it is interesting to note that not all high-fibre foods are low on the Glycaemic Index - the index that measures how quickly foods are absorbed into the bloodstream. For example, baked potatoes, parsnips, whole wheat bread and dates (which all feature regularly in the F-plan Diet) are high on the index and quickly absorbed into the bloodstream. The diet works like any diet - by reducing the total number of calories that are eaten.

What is dietary fibre?

Previously called 'roughage', dietary fibre is the term that describes the carbohydrates that human's can't digest. Dietary fibre is found in plant foods such as cereals, pulses, fruits and vegetables and occurs mainly in the plant cell wall where it provides structural support for the plant.

What's the link with weight loss?

Most high-fibre plans for weight loss still come with a reduction in calories. The F-Plan diet, for example, recommended a calorie restriction of between 850-1,500 calories a day – and of course, it's this calorie restriction that helps you lose weight. However, there are many reasons why including more fibre in your diet can help boost weight loss and make slimming less painful.

To start with, unlike other carbohydrates, most dietary fibre doesn't provide any calories. This means fibre-rich foods are often lower in energy than foods containing no fibre or only small amounts, making them ideal for people who are trying to lose weight.

Secondly, high fibre foods generally take longer to chew. As well as helping you to feel more satisfied when you eat, this automatically slows down the speed at which you eat, giving your brain time to register feelings of fullness so that you're less like to overeat. But that's not the only way fibre-rich foods help to control appetite. Fibre acts like a sponge and absorbs and holds on to water as its chewed in the mouth and passes into the stomach. This means fibre-rich foods swell up in your stomach and this can help to fill you up. Better still, fibre stays in the stomach for longer as it's harder to digest and this helps to keep you feeling fuller for longer, so you're less likely to want to snack in between meals.

So how much fibre should I eat a day to lose weight and how much can I expect to lose?

Regardless of whether you want to lose weight or maintain your weight, the Department of Health recommends adults eat an average of 18g of fibre a day with a range of 12-24g. If you want to lose weight, you'll still need to restrict your calorie intake as recommended by Weight Loss Resources and the amount you can expect to lose will depend entirely on the degree of this restriction. Weight Loss Resources recommends you aim to lose no more than 2lb a week, although you might lose slightly more in the first few weeks when your body loses water as well as fat. This follows the guidelines recommended by nutrition experts.

Has a high-fibre diet got any other health benefits?

Definitely. Having spent a long time in the stomach, fibre moves through the large intestine relatively quickly and health experts believe this helps to keep the digestive system healthy, preventing bowel problems such as constipation, diverticular disease and haemorrhoids (piles), as well as reducing the risk of bowel cancer. Interestingly, all these conditions tend to be uncommon in undeveloped countries where intakes of fibre are high, compared to Western societies where these medical problems are widespread and fibre intakes are low.

Furthermore, most fibre-rich foods are also low in fat and packed with vitamins and minerals – and when it comes to preventing disease, it seems that it's this whole package of nutrients that's important. For example, wholegrains like wheat, barley, oats, rye and rice contain not just fibre, but a number of nutrients that may reduce the risk of heart disease, stroke, certain cancers and diabetes by as much as 30 per cent. These include antioxidant nutrients vitamin E, zinc and selenium and a range of plant compounds called phytochemicals.

I'd heard that a high-fibre intake was good for my heart. What's the link?

Several large studies in America, Finland and Norway have found that people who eat relatively large amounts of wholegrain cereals have significantly lower rates of heart disease and stroke. It's thought that a particular type of fibre called soluble fibre may be partly responsible as it helps to lower blood cholesterol levels.

Tell me more about soluble fibre?

Dietary fibre can be divided into two main types – soluble and insoluble fibre. Soluble fibre is thought to bind with cholesterol and prevent it from being reabsorbed into the bloodstream. This lowers the amount of cholesterol in the blood, therefore reducing the risk of heart disease. But that's not all. Soluble fibre also forms a gel in the intestine, which is thought to slow down the digestion and absorption of carbohydrates, especially glucose. This means it can help to keep blood sugar levels steady, preventing feelings of hunger that leave you reaching for the biscuit tin. Foods rich in soluble fibre include fruits, vegetables, oats, barley, and pulses such as beans, lentils and peas.

In contrast, insoluble fibre helps to keep the digestive system in good working order by increasing the bulk and softness of the stools, which in turn assists the smooth passage of food through the body. It's this type of fibre that helps to prevent bowel complaints like constipation and cancer. Foods rich in insoluble fibre include wholemeal flour and bread, wholegrain breakfast cereals, bran, brown rice, wholemeal pasta, grains and some fruits and vegetables.

Eating a range of fibre-rich foods, rather than just one or two sources, is the best way to ensure you get a mixture of both soluble and insoluble fibre – and make the most of the health benefits offered by both.

So is a high-fibre diet suitable for people with diabetes?

Yes, health experts recommend that people with diabetes have a good intake of fibre in the same way as the rest of the population. But it's always wise to speak to your doctor or dietician before making any changes to your diet, especially if you are on medication such as tablets or insulin.

What about high-fibre intakes for children?

Although older children and teenagers will benefit from eating plenty of fibre-rich foods, very young children shouldn't be given large amounts. This is because they have small tummies and generally consume much smaller quantities of food than older children and adults. Because fibre-rich foods tend to be filling but reasonably low in energy, young children may not be able to satisfy their energy requirements and this may mean they don't grow as well as they should.

Is it still possible to get enough fibre if I follow a wheat-free diet?

Yes, providing you include plenty of fruit, veg, pulses and brown rice. See the chart here to see how you can make up 18g of fibre a day using non-wheat foods.

Is there a link with fibre and the glycaemic index of a food?

Yes. Generally speaking, the more fibre a food contains the lower its glycaemic index will be. This is because fibre acts as a physical barrier and slows down the absorption of carbohydrates into the blood.

Are there any cons to high fibre diets?

Wind is the main problem! Some fibre is fermented in the large intestine by bacteria that live there and this results in the production of gases like methane, hydrogen and carbon dioxide. The amount of gas produced depends on the type of fibre eaten and the gut bacteria present. But it explains why some slimmers find that excessive wind, discomfort and bloating occur if they suddenly boost their fibre intake to help them lose weight.

Fortunately, this is usually a short-lived problem as the large intestine and gut bacteria gradually adapt to an increased intake of fibre. That's why it's important to introduce fibre-rich foods into the diet gradually – and to persevere with them.

Constipation can also be a side effect of a high-fibre diet if fluid intake isn't also increased. This is because fibre acts like a sponge and absorbs water. The easiest way to avoid this, is to boost fluid intakes together with fibre intakes.

Fruit, vegetables, nuts, seeds and pulses are all good sources of fibre. But with cereal-based foods such as breakfast cereals, pasta, rice and bread, the amount of fibre depends on how much of the outer layer of the grain has been stripped away in the milling and refining process. The more processing a cereal has been through, the lower its fibre content will be. Meanwhile, it's not just fibre that's lost during processing. Many vitamins and minerals are also found in the outer layers of the grain, so when these are removed, these vitamins and minerals are also lost. As a golden rule, always choose brown over white. When it comes to shopping, this means bagels, croissants, cornflakes and white rice should stay on the shelf, while wholegrain bread, wholewheat pasta, branflakes and brown rice should go into the trolley.

The following foods are all good sources of dietary fibre…

- Wholemeal, granary and softgrain varieties of bread
- Jacket potatoes, new potatoes in their skins and baked potato skins
- Wholegrain breakfast cereals, eg. Weetabix, branflakes, unsweetened muesli, Shreddies and porridge oats
- Wholemeal pasta and brown rice
- Beans, lentils and peas
- Fresh and dried fruits – particularly if the skins are eaten
- Vegetables – particularly if the skins are eaten
- Nuts and seeds
- Wholemeal flour

How about adding bran to my breakfast cereal?

Bran is a rich source of fibre, but there are far more pleasurable and healthy ways to boost fibre intakes! Not only is raw bran quite unpalatable but it doesn't provide the other nutrients found in fibre-rich foods such as wholemeal bread and wholegrain cereals. Plus it can reduce the absorption of certain nutrients such as iron, calcium and zinc. For this reason, it's no longer recommended that you sprinkle raw bran onto breakfast cereal.

Is there a simple way to tell if a food is a good source of fibre?

Looking at food labels is one of the easiest ways to identify whether or not a food contains a little or a lot of fibre. The Food Standards Agency recommends that any product claiming to be a 'source' of fibre should contain 3g fibre per 100g or at least 3g of fibre in the amount that could reasonably be expected to be eaten in one day. To claim that a food is high in fibre, the product must contain at least 6g per 100g or at least 6g in the amount that could be expected to be eaten each day. Otherwise, use the table below to see the fibre content of some common foods.

Sources of Dietary Fibre

As well as including plenty of fibre-rich foods, this chart also includes some low-fibre foods so you can see how they compare. To increase dietary fibre, as a general rule, swap white foods for brown foods and aim for an intake of 18g of fibre a day.

Food	Serving Sizes	Dietary Fibre Content (g)
Breakfast Cereals		
All-bran	6tbsp	10.3
Shredded Wheat	2	4.4
Branflakes	4tbsp	4.2
Weetabix	2	3.9
Unsweetened muesli	3tbsp	3.4
Fruit 'n' fibre	4tbsp	2.2
Porridge	1 bowl	1.3
Cornflakes	5tbsp	0.3
Bread		
Wholemeal bread	1 slice	2.1
Granary bread	1 slice	1.5
Brown bread	1 slice	1.3
White bread	1 slice	0.5
Cooked pasta and rice		
Wholewheat pasta	230g	8.1
White pasta	230g	2.8
Brown rice	180g	1.4
White rice	180g	0.2
Fruit		
Avocado	1/2 small	3.4
Dried apricots	6	3

Orange	1	2.7
Apple	1	1.8
Peach	1	1.7
Banana	1	1.1
Strawberries	100g	1.1
Grapes	100g	0.7
Vegetables		
Baked beans	1 small can (200g)	7.4
Jacket potato	1 medium (180g)	4.9
Frozen peas	3 tbsp (90g)	4.6
Broccoli	85g	2
Green beans	90g	1.7
Red Lentils	3 tbsp (90g)	1.7
Cabbage	95g	1.7
Carrots	60g	1.5
Cauliflower	90g	1.4
Sweetcorn	3 tbsp (90g)	1.3
Tomato	1	0.9
Lettuce	30g	0.3
Nuts and seeds		
Roasted and salted peanuts	50g bag	3
Almonds	6 whole	1
Sunflower seeds	1tbsp	1
Peanut butter	1tbsp	0.8
Brazil nuts	3 whole	0.4

NB: Serving sizes are based on medium portions.

Fat Flush

The Fat Flush Plan is both a detox diet and a weight loss diet. The idea is to provide all the necessary ingredients to boost metabolism, reduce water retention, and promote fat loss.

The program has 3 phases:

Phase 1 (2 weeks)
This is a restrictive phase of between 1100-1200 calories per day. The intention here is to "lose bloat" - which refers to reducing water retention *as well as* some fat loss. In this phase you are *not allowed* to eat; margarine, alcohol, sugar, oils or fats (except flaxseed oil), grains, bread, cereal, starchy vegetables, dairy products. Even the herbs and spices are restricted to a small list.

Phase 2 (Ongoing)
Here the calorie allowance is lifted - to 1200-1500 calories. The idea is to continue on with the program until the desired weight loss is achieved.

Phase 3 (The maintenance phase)
Essentially a weight maintenance phase, with a caloric intake of 1500 calories or over. Some starchy carbs are gradually re-introduced, along with gluten-free grains, and some dairy.

Exercise
The program contains a significant exercise component. This can be anything from 20 to 40 minutes of exercise per day, depending on the phase. This is typically low-impact (walking). Strength training (lifting weights) is also on the list (twice a week). A sleep prescription of exactly 8 hours per night is also required.

Sample Meal Plan - Fat Flush Phase 1

Upon Waking
"Long Life" cocktail [psyllium husks in cran-water]

Before Breakfast
8 oz hot water with lemon juice

Breakfast
Vegetable scramble - 2 scrambled eggs, with spinach, green peppers, scallions, and parsley.
8 oz glass of cran-water [diluted unsweetened cranberry juice]

Snack
1/2 Large grapefruit
20 minutes before lunch
8 oz glass of cran water

Lunch
4 ounces of salmon with lemon and garlic, warm asparagus, mixed-green salad with broccoli florets and cucumber, 1 tablespoon flaxseed oil, and one 8 oz glass of cran-water

Mid afternoon snack
2 8 oz glass cran-water

4pm Snack
1 apple

20 minutes before dinner
8 oz glass of cran water

Dinner
4 ounces of grilled lamb chop with pinch of cinnamon and dried mustard, sautéed kale in broth, baked summer squash with a touch of cloves, and 1 tablespoon flaxseed oil

Mid evening
"Long life" cocktail

Fat Flush Pros and Cons

The Up side
The Fat Flush program has all the elements of a good and healthy weight loss program. It isn't hard to find success stories regarding this program (however the true test is always the test of time - is the fat loss sustained or temporary?).
Remember this diet is a *detox* or *cleansing* diet, thus the very restrictive phase one. Unless healthy eating patterns are applied to your lifestyle, any benefits gained will soon be lost.

The Down side
One criticism is that the calorie level in Phase 1 may be too low for some people (particularly men), and the lower calorie levels could have the affect of slowing down metabolism rather than speeding it up.
There is a significant exercise portion (which is a good thing) and fortunately the longer exercise is added during phase 3. However there is little chance the calorie levels of phase 1 (or 2) will support a strong exercise regimen.
This diet is like many other diet books - the one size fits all approach will never suit everyone. Eight hours a sleep a night may be excellent for some, but with 40 minutes brisk walking a day, plus 2 weights sessions per week, this sleep is simply not enough for some people.

Fit For Life

The Fit for Life Diet originated in the 1980s in a book written by Harvey and Marilyn Diamond. Basically it is a food-combining weight-loss diet that has two basic tenets:
1) It's not what you eat but when you eat and how you combine your food that determines weight loss and health.
2) Always eat fruit alone, never with other foods. The Diamonds maintain that following these tenets will lead to weight reduction and increased energy levels.
They further claim that the body experiences three digestive cycles during the day: appropriation, which is eating and digesting (noon to 8 p.m.); assimilation, which is absorption and the use of nutrients (8 p.m. to 4 a.m.); and elimination of body wastes (4 a.m. to noon). According to the Fit for Life Diet theory, by eating foods in the right combination at the right times, following these natural cycles, the body can rid itself of toxins and excess weight.

How Fit for Life Diet Works

According to the Diamonds, combining certain foods is at a meal is undesirable. Any food besides fruits and vegetables is considered a "concentrated food" (having a low water content), and concentrated foods cannot be combined with one another. Fruit must be eaten alone. For example, a typical day's menu would begin with only fruit or fruit juice before noon. For lunch and dinner you can either have a carbohydrate-based meal, which would be grains, beans, and vegetables, or a protein-based meal, which would be protein and vegetables. A fruit snack is allowed after dinner, but only if you wait at least three hours after eating dinner. Fruits are okay during the day because of their high water content, which washes and cleanses the body of toxins. However, if fruit is eaten at the end of a meal, it ferments and causes digestion and weight problems. According to the Diamonds, actually drinking water with a meal can be debilitating.

Advantages of Fit for Life Diet
- The Fit for Life Diet encourages dieters to eat lots of fruits and vegetables.
- You can eat as much of the specific foods you want, since there is never a reason to measure portions or worry about counting calories or grams of fat.

Disadvantages of Fit for Life Diet
- In reality, the Fit for Life Diet isn't all that simple since you can't eat fruits with other foods, and you must not combine proteins and starches.
- Dieters who are into the meat-potato-vegetable routine are in for some dramatic changes.

Dieticians Comments About Fit for Life Diet
The idea of food combining has been around since the turn of the century, and is relatively outdated. The Fit for Life Diet theories are, for the most part, unsupported by scientific or clinical evidence. For example, the Fit for Life Diet premise that we cannot digest a combination of foods has no scientific validity whatsoever. Nutritionists say the human digestive system has the enzymes and other conditions necessary for digesting and absorbing an extremely wide range of foods, whether eaten in isolation or in combinations. Human beings are naturally omnivorous and we can eat grain foods, vegetables, fruits, meat, fish, and dairy products (among many other foods) and thrive on a huge variety of combinations of foods.
With regard to their advice not to combine foods, it is actually quite difficult to avoid combining proteins with carbohydrates. The Diamonds seem to be unaware that the "carbohydrate foods"

bread, potatoes, rice, spaghetti, and legumes (foods such as beans, peas, soy products and lentils) also contain significant quantities of protein. Eating these foods on their own (which they regard as appropriate) constitutes the very act of food-combining that they seem to think will cause indigestion.

The Fit for Life diet is based on a Four-Week Detoxification Process, with menus based on the Energy Ladder. The weight loss program recommends purchasing a juicer because fresh fruit and vegetable juices are a central component to this diet.

Energy Ladder

A.M.
Fresh Fruit and Fruit Juices
Fresh Vegetables Juice and Salads
Steamed Vegetables, Raw Nuts & Seeds
Grains, Breads, Potatoes, Legumes
Meat, Chicken, Fish, Dairy

P.M.
The energy ladder indicates which goods to early in the day and which to eat later. Food closest to the A.M can be eaten anytime of the day, but those closest to the P.M. should not be eaten early in the day. Any day on which fruits and vegetables are all you consume will be a high energy, maximum weight-loss day.

Breakfast
Breakfast under the Fit for Life diet is always the same. Until noon everyday you may have as much fresh fruit juice and fresh fruit as you desire. Try to start each day with a fresh fruit juice - orange, apple, tangerine, melon, or pineapple are preferred. It is recommended that you have several pieces of fruit. One serving of fruit is the amount that leaves you feeling comfortable
  - Start your day with Fresh Fruit juice if you desire, recommended quantity: eight to fourteen ounces
  - Throughout the morning have pieces of fruit as you feel hungry
  - Have a minimum of two servings of fruit as you feel hungry
  - Your maximum fruit intake should be governed by your needs. Have as much as you desire. Do not undereat or overeat fruit
  - Eat melons before other fruit
  - Eat bananas when are particularly hunger and are craving heavier food

Main-Course Salad
The diet also emphasizes the main-course salad approach to eating. The concept insures that the largest portion of what you are eating is fresh, live vegetables. Whatever you have added to your salad, the bulk of your meal will break down more quickly and pass through your system more easily due to its properly combined nature and the presence of all the fresh raw vegetables. The book includes recipes for several main-course salads, but feel free to create your own.

A Day in Fit for Life diet
(sample menu plan based on the Energy Ladder)
  - Breakfast: Always the same (see above)
  - Lunch: 4-8 ounces of fresh carrot juice, energy salad

- Dinner: Harvest Soup, Hot Buttered Corn Tortillas, Teriyaki Broccoli, Tangy Green Coleslaw

Food Combining

Food-combining diets first came to prominence with the Hay Diet in the 1930s, and have gained popularity in recent years. There are several food-combining diets on the market, such as the popular Fit for Life Diet. Food-combining diets are generally based on the theory that in order to optimize digestion and weight loss, specific foods are to be eaten at certain times and eaten in the following combinations:

- Proteins (beans, nuts, seeds, meat, fish, and poultry) and carbohydrates (grains, pasta, breads, cereal, rice, carrots, etc.) should be eaten at separate meals. However, proteins can be eaten with vegetables and starches can be combined with vegetables.
- Fruits should be eaten alone.
- Dairy products are prohibited, as are some other food products depending on the particular type of diet.

Some versions advocate eating only fruit or fruit juices before noon, and focus on other types of food for the remainder of the day. A typical food-combining diet lasts for five weeks, although some versions are indefinite.

How Food Combining Diets Work

Digestive enzymes are secreted in very specific amounts and at very specific times. Different food types require different digestive secretions. Carbohydrate foods require carbohydrate-splitting enzymes, whereas protein foods require protein-splitting enzymes. The rules for food combining are briefly explained below.

Advantages of Food-Combining Diets

- Food-combining diets encourage eating fruits and vegetables.
- A food-combining diet may benefit you for a couple of days, as a type of detox diet.

Disadvantages of Food Combining Diets

- Food-combining diets can be difficult and time-consuming to follow. Favourite pairings, such as chicken with potatoes, tofu with rice, soy-milk fruit shakes, beans and rice, and tuna sandwiches are not allowed.
- Lacking firm scientific basis, many food-combining diets provide inadequate vitamins and minerals. Protein and carbohydrates cannot be eaten together, so people have to choose one or the other. As a result, people often consume more carbohydrates than protein, as carbohydrates tend to be more filling and satisfying. Special care should be taken to ensure adequate intake of protein, calcium, zinc, vitamin D, and vitamin B12.

Dieticians Comments About Food-Combining Diets

Although food-combining diets have helped a number of people with dietary and weight loss problems, there is no hard scientific evidence to support the theory behind these diets. Nutritionists say the idea that weight loss is more likely if you separate certain foods is completely without foundation. In fact, many health practitioners believe that combining protein and carbohydrates can be beneficial. When protein and fats are combined with carbohydrates, the absorption of carbohydrates is slowed. This helps to maintain stable blood sugar and insulin levels and prevent cravings.

Sample Food Combining Menu

The essence of a food combining meal plan is ensure that starches and proteins should never be combined in the same meal. Here is a sample meal plan for a Food Combining diet:

Breakfast:
- Two slices of toast with butter and shredded cheddar cheese
- Cup of herbal tea

Lunch:
- Baked potato with sour cream and chives

Dinner:
- Broiled salmon with three-bean salad
- Small glass of red wine

Snacks:
- Tropical fruit salad: pineapple, mango, raspberry and kiwi

Glycemic Index (GI Diet)

The G.I. Diet developed by Rick Gallop, former president of the Heart and Stroke Foundation of Ontario, offers a unique diet program based on the Glycemic Index (GI). The theory behind the diet is that foods with a low GI value slowly release sugar into the blood, providing you with a steady supply of energy. This gives you a more satisfied feeling so that you're less likely to snack. In contrast, foods with a high GI value cause a rapid—but short-lived—rise in blood sugar. This leaves you lacking in energy and feeling hungry within a short time, causing you to eat more food. If this pattern is frequently repeated, you're likely to gain weight as a result of constantly overeating.

Most high-GI foods, such as those made from white flour are heavily processed and the essential nutrients have been stripped away. Conversely, low-GI foods, such as fruits, vegetables, nuts, legumes, whole grains, lean meat/fish, and low-fat dairy are rich in nutrients essential for your good health.

How it Works

With the G.I. Diet, foods are classified according to how quickly they are absorbed into the system, helping you recognize which foods will make you feel fuller for longer. This program is easy to follow, as the G.I. Diet makes all the calculations for you by organizing all the foods in one of three categories: red light foods, which you avoid if you want to lose weight; yellow light foods that can be eaten occasionally; and green light foods that can be eaten as much as you like.

Green light foods are essentially fruits and vegetables. The yellow light foods, such as bananas and steak, can be eaten once in a while and in moderation. And the red light foods, such as pizza, bagels, and bacon, are the ones people should stay away from if they want to lose weight.

Advantages
- The G.I. Diet is not only good for losing weight, but has been found to reduce "bad" LDL cholesterol.
- Unlike the Atkins Diet, which bans most carbohydrates, especially in the early stages, the G.I. diet, actively encourages you to eat many carbohydrates and antioxidant-rich fruits and vegetables.

Disadvantages
- One of the main limitations of the G.I. Diet is the fact that it's difficult to estimate the GI value of a meal.
- You might experience nutritional deficiencies from not eating higher-GI foods.

Dieticians Comments About G.I. Diet

In general, most nutritionists are supportive of the basic principles of the G.I. Diet. The diet generally contains plenty of fruit and vegetables, and recommends eating fewer refined carbohydrates. They do, however, believe that many popular diet authors have taken a controversial nutritional concept—the Glycemic Index—out of the context for which it was intended: as a guideline for diabetics.

Also, critics contend the diet's color-coding system only identifies the effect different foods have on blood sugar levels when they are eaten on their own and, consequently, many believe this is one of the main problems with the G.I. Diet. Basically, when you eat foods together, as in a meal, the GI value of that whole meal is reflected in portion sizes and the individual GI values for each food eaten. As a guideline, the more low-GI foods you include in a meal, the lower the overall GI value for that meal. For instance, mashed potatoes have a high GI value, but if the meal includes pan-seared salmon, a big salad, and steamed broccoli-all of which have low GI values-these foods will minimize the impact on blood sugar levels that come from eating the potatoes.

Breakfast
Cereal with Seeds, Walnuts and Fruit [Calories 290]
1 Shredded Wheat biscuit
1/2 cup non-fat milk
1 tbsp pumpkin seeds
4 chopped walnuts
1 apple, chopped
Cover wheat biscuit with the milk and top with seeds, chopped nuts and apple.

Snack Suggestion
1 orange [Calories 70]

Lunch
Grilled Ham & Swiss on Rye and Fruit [Calories 340]
1 slice rye bread or whole wheat bread
1 oz low-fat Swiss cheese
3 oz deli ham
1/2 tsp honey mustard
4 cherry tomatoes
1 kiwi fruit
1. Toast the bread on one side, under broiler. Spread the non-toasted side with the mustard.
2. Put ham on top, and cover with cheese. Broil until cheese melts.

Snack Suggestion
Low-fat yogurt, handful of walnuts or almonds [100]

Dinner
Broiled Chicken Breast, Lentils and Vegetables [Calories 344]
5 oz skinless, boneless, chicken breast
1/2 cup cooked lentils
1 cup fresh or frozen broccoli
1 cup fresh or frozen green beans
1. Spray the chicken with cooking spray and broil until tender.
2. Serve with the cooked lentils and steamed or microwave vegetables.
Extra Daily Allowance
1/2 cup fat-free milk (or equivalent)

Total Daily Calories: 1189
Your daily meals on this diet contain an average of 1200 calories. Depending on your gender and how much weight you have to lose, you may increase this to 2000+ calories, by choosing from a wide range of calorie-controlled snacks.

The Grapefruit Diet

This diet is based on the premise that grapefruit has fat burning properties. The grapefruit diet lasts 12 days, but if an individual wants to continue they must take at least two days off before doing so. While there is no hard evidence that grapefruit burns fat, the diet does have some success stories.

Most meals are accompanied by grapefruit. It is also recommended that participants drink about 8 glasses of water per day. This regimented diet does not allow most complex carbs, and doesn't allow for snacking in between meals. However, the consumption of most vegetables is encouraged and you are allowed to prepare them in generous amounts of butter.

For breakfast, a typical meal involves half a grapefruit, eggs, bacon, and coffee or tea to drink. An example of a lunch and dinner involve grapefruit (naturally), salad, and meat of any style and amount. This is a very low calorie diet, and people often report dizziness and a lack of energy.

Version 1
Breakfast
Half a grapefruit (or 8 ounces grapefruit juice)
2 eggs any style
2 slices of bacon

Lunch
Half a grapefruit (or 8 ounces grapefruit juice)
Salad with any dressing Meat (any style in any amount)

Dinner
Half a grapefruit (or 8 ounces grapefruit juice)
Salad with dressing (or green vegetable cooked in butter)
Meat or fish (any style, cooked any way)
Black coffee or tea

Bedtime Snack
8 ounces of tomato juice (or 8 ounces of skim milk)

Rules:
1. Drink 64 ounces of water a day (eight 8 ounce glasses)
2. At any meal you may eat until you are full.
3. You must eat the minimum listed at each meal.
4. You cannot eliminate anything from the diet.
5. Cut down on coffee, it affects the insulin balance.
6. Don't eat between meals.
7. You can fry food in butter.
8. Do not eat desserts, breads, and white vegetables or sweet potatoes.
9. You may double or triple helpings of meat, salad or vegetables.
10. Eat until you are stuffed. The more you eat the more weight you will lose.
11. Stay on the diet 12 days, then stop the diet for 2 days and repeat.

Version 2
Breakfast
Half a grapefruit
Black coffee

Lunch
Half a grapefruit
1 Egg Salad
1 slice of bread, toasted
Black coffee

Dinner
Half a grapefruit
2 Eggs
Half a head of lettuce
Tomato
1 slice of bread, toasted
Black tea or coffee

Hamptons Diet

The Hamptons Diet is a low-carbohydrate diet developed by Dr. Fred Pescatore, former medical director of the Atkins Centre. The basic premise of the Hamptons Diet is to eat more vegetables, fish, and omega-3 fatty acids, and to consume most of your fats in the form of monounsaturated fats, a premise shared by the Mediterranean Diet.

Central to the Hamptons Diet is the secret ingredient macadamia nut oil, which Pescatore claims to be "the most monounsaturated oil on the planet." This oil is basically used for everything from salad dressings to marinades and even for cooking. The oils in macadamia are 84% monounsaturated, 3.5% polyunsaturated, and 12.5% saturated. The monounsaturated portion contains oleic fatty acid plus the highest known level of paimitoleic fatty acid, which is also present in beneficial fish oils, and may be nutritionally significant.

How Hamptons Diet Works

In addition to promoting the consumption of the right kind of fats, the Hamptons Diet also advises to avoid processed foods, which are the foods that promote chronic diseases like diabetes, cancer, obesity, and heart disease. Processed foods often contain trans-fatty acids, the ones now related to cancer more than saturated fats. Manufactured, brand-name foods are not considered healthy foods. The way to eat healthy is to purchase ingredients in bulk, like vegetables, fresh meats, and fruits, then prepare them yourself. Where possible, the food should be organic. With the right recipes, you don't need to be a chef to make healthy meals fast.

Advantages of Hamptons Diet

- The Hamptons Diet, unlike other low-carbohydrate diets, does not promote the consumption of unhealthy fats like animal fat (saturated fat), hydrogenated oils, and soybean oil, which is high in omega-6 fatty acids.

Disadvantages of Hamptons Diet

- Ingredients are so upscale you need to be able to afford to live in the Hamptons to afford this diet.

Dieticians Comments About Hamptons Diet

As far as popular low-carbohydrate diets go, the Hamptons Diet seems to have some sensible advice—particularly compared with the Atkins Diet. The diet encourages dieters to shift to a more balanced range of foods including monounsaturated fats, complex carbohydrates, and no processed foods, which is a step in the right direction. However, nutritionists believe it cuts way back on healthful foods like fruits, vegetables, and dairy. On the flip side, unlike other low-carbohydrate diets that encourage the widespread consumption of saturated fats, the Hamptons Diet places a lot of emphasis on consuming the right kind of fats-specifically monounsaturated fats.

Day 1 Sample Menu Plan

Breakfast
Goat Cheese and Arugula Omelette
Yield: 2 servings Carbohydrates per serving: 4
This will serve as your basic omelette recipe. You can substitute your favourite ingredients — as

long as they're on your acceptable list — for the goat cheese and the arugula listed here.

Ingredients

4 eggs

2 tablespoons water

2 tablespoons heavy cream

Salt

Pepper

1 tablespoon grated parmesan cheese

1 tablespoon macadamia nut oil

2 large handfuls of arugula leaves, fresh from your garden

1/2 cup crumbled goat cheese

Directions

Whisk all the ingredients, except the goat cheese and the arugula, together in a bowl until frothy. Heat the oil in a skillet until hot. Sauté the arugula for 1 minute or until wilted. Pour the egg mixture over the greens and, as they begin to set, lift the edge of the eggs with a spatula to allow the liquid eggs to slide beneath the cooked eggs. Continue to cook over a low heat until the eggs are set but not too firm. Before they set too much, simply add the goat cheese or whatever other ingredient you choose. Fold the omelette in half and serve.

Lunch

Roast Beef with Melted Provolone Roll-Ups

Ingredients

1 pound thinly sliced roast beef

4 slices provolone cheese

Horseradish

Salt and pepper to taste

Directions

On a cookie sheet, divide the roast beef into 4 equal portions. Lay a slice of provolone cheese onto each bed of roast beef and spread with horseradish. Sprinkle with salt and pepper. Roll up, and secure with toothpicks that have been sitting in a water bath for 30 minutes. Place in a preheated 375-degree F oven until the cheese melts, about 5 to 8 minutes, and serve.

Green Salad with choice of dressing (Sherry Vinaigrette, Sour Cream Dressing, Creamy Peanut Dressing)

Dinner

Creole Rubbed Tuna Steak

Yield: 4 servings Carbohydrates per serving: 0

This takes advance preparation time.

Ingredients

4 (8-ounce) tuna fillets

1 tablespoon curry powder

4 tablespoons macadamia nut oil

2 tablespoons minced fresh garlic

1 Scotch bonnet pepper, stemmed, seeded, and minced

1 teaspoon grated fresh ginger

Sea salt

Freshly ground coarse black pepper

Arugula leaves (raw)

Directions

Combine all the ingredients except arugula in a stainless steel bowl, and mix together until the tuna steaks are well coated. Refrigerate for 2 hours. On a preheated grill over high heat, sear the tuna on each side for 2 minutes. This will leave the tuna seared on the outside but raw on the inside. For more doneness, cook on each side for an additional minute until it reaches the desired temperature. Serve over a bed of arugula leaves.

Gardiner's Zucchini Salad

Yield: 6 servings Carbohydrates per serving: 6

This recipe requires advance preparation.

Ingredients

2 pounds zucchini, mix of yellow and green

1/2 red onion, thinly sliced

1 (4-ounce) can mild green chillies, drained and diced

4 ounces your favourite olives, sliced

Oil and vinegar dressing

1 avocado, chopped

1/2 cup queso fresco

Directions

Cut the zucchini crosswise into 1/2-inch slices. Cover with water in a saucepan and bring to a boil, reduce heat, and cook about 4 minutes or until just barely tender. Drain, and refresh in cold water. Do not overcook. Drain again. In a stainless steel bowl, combine the zucchini, onion, chillies, and olives; mix with oil and vinegar dressing, and chill at least 2 hours. Before serving, mix in the avocado, and top with the crumbled cheese.

Raspberries and Crème Fraiche

Ingredients

1/2 cup raspberries

Crème fraiche

Snack

Directions

Green and red pepper strips with choice of dipping sauce (Spinach Avocado Dip, Pesto Dip, Cilantro Nut Dip)

Dressings & Dips

Sherry Vinaigrette

Ingredients

3 tablespoons Dijon mustard

1 egg yolk

4 teaspoons sherry vinegar

3/4 cup macadamia nut oil

Salt

Pepper

Directions

In a mixing bowl, whisk together the mustard and the egg yolk. Whisk in 1 teaspoon of the vinegar, then slowly whisk in the oil to make a thick emulsion. Whisk in the rest of the vinegar, and season with salt and pepper.

Creamy Peanut Dressing

Yield: 4 servings Carbohydrates per serving: 2

Ingredients

2 tablespoons Mayonnaise

2 tablespoons heavy cream

1 teaspoon Dijon mustard

1 teaspoon horseradish

1 tablespoon crunchy, unsweetened peanut butter

Directions

Mix all ingredients together in a small food processor until smooth.

Sour Cream Dressing

Yield: 8 servings Carbohydrates per serving: 2

Ingredients

3 hard-cooked eggs

Juice of 1 lemon, freshly squeezed

1 cup sour cream

2 tablespoons heavy cream

Salt

Pepper

Directions

Put the egg yolks and the rest of the ingredients in a food processor, and pulse until smooth. You may thin it with extra cream to gain the desired consistency.

Cilantro Nut Dip

Yield: 24 servings Carbohydrates per serving: 1

Ingredients

1 cup chopped fresh cilantro

1/4 cup fresh grated parmesan cheese

1/2 cup chopped macadamia nuts

2 cloves garlic, minced

8 ounces smooth goat cheese

1/4 cup macadamia nut oil

Kosher salt to taste

Directions

Combine all the ingredients except the oil in a food processor, and pulse until well combined. Gradually add in the oil, processing until smooth. This can even be used on meats and fish — it is that rich.

Spinach Avocado Dip

Yield: 24 servings Carbohydrates per serving: 1

Ingredients
2 cups fresh spinach leaves
1/4 cup heavy cream
1/2 red onion, finely diced
1 tablespoon green chillies
1 teaspoon fresh-squeezed lime juice
1/4 cup fresh chopped cilantro
1/2 medium avocado, peeled and sliced

Directions
Cook the spinach in a pot of boiling salted water for about 1 minute. Drain, and rinse under cold water; drain again, and squeeze dry. Put the remaining ingredients except the avocado in a food processor, and pulse until the spinach is finely chopped, but don't over blend. Mash the avocado separately, then stir into the spinach mixture.

Pesto Dip
Yield: 12 servings Carbohydrates per serving: 1
Ingredients
1/4 cup fresh pesto
1 teaspoon lime juice, freshly squeezed
1/2 cup Mayonnaise
1/4 teaspoon salt
1/8 teaspoon freshly ground black pepper
1 tablespoon toasted pine nuts

Directions
Combine all the ingredients except the nuts in a bowl, and season with salt and pepper. Transfer to a serving bowl, and sprinkle with pine nuts.

Hay System

The Hay Diet created by Dr. William Hay, is known as a "food-combining diet" and is based on the premise of not mixing proteins with carbohydrates. This in turn aids digestion and facilitates weight loss, and keeps the digestive system healthy. This conclusion was drawn from the fact that the eating habits of our ancestors were not as complex as they are today, and since we evolved from them, changing our eating habits to those of our ancestors will reduce unwanted gains in body fat as seen in the age of the caveman.

How it Works

The Hay Diet consists of six basic rules:

Starches and sugars should not be eaten with proteins or acid fruits at the same meal.

Vegetables, salads, and fruits (whether acid or sweet), if correctly combined, should form the major part of the diet.

Proteins, starches, and fats should be eaten only in small quantities.

Eat only whole grains and unprocessed starches, and exclude refined, processed foods such as white flour, white sugar, and margarine.

Allow at least four hours between meals of different types.

Milk does not combine well with food and should be kept to a minimum.

Advantages

- The Hay Diet can reverse chronic and degenerative conditions such as constipation, indigestion and arthritis.
- It can be beneficial to asthma and allergy sufferers.

Disadvantages

- The Hay Diet can be hard to follow as there are many complicated charts outlining the do's and don'ts.
- Lacking firm scientific basis, many food-combining diets provide inadequate vitamins and minerals. Protein and carbohydrates cannot be eaten together, so people have to choose one or the other. As a result, people often consume more carbohydrates than protein, as carbohydrates tend to be more filling and satisfying. Special care should be taken to ensure adequate intake of protein, calcium, zinc, vitamin D, and vitamin B12.

Dieticians Comments About Hay Diet

The Hay Diet first gained credence as a method of weight loss since most dietary restrictions usually mean consuming fewer calories than the body needs. Hence it is no better than any other diet that is low in calories.

Scientifically, the Hay Diet is impossible to achieve since most starchy foods, such as bread and potatoes, contain some protein. The body is well adapted to digest both proteins and starch, and the enzymes necessary to digest them are secreted in response to the food being in the stomach.

Hay rules

- Starches and sugars **should not be eaten** with proteins and acid fruits at the same meal.
- Vegetables, salads and fruits (whether acid or sweet) if correctly combined should form the major part of the diet.
- Proteins, starches and fats should be eaten in small quantities.
- Only whole grains and unprocessed starches should be used and all refined and processed foods should be eliminated from the diet.

- Not less than four hours between starch and protein meals.
- Milk does not combine well with food and should be kept to a minimum.

Don't mix foods that fight, so in the below lists don't mix anything from list 1 with list 3.
1. Proteins: All meat, poultry, eggs, dairy, cheese, eggs, fish, soya beans yoghurt,
2. Neutral: Most vegetables (except potatoes and artichokes), seeds, all salads, nuts, herbs, cream, olive oil
3. Carbohydrate: Biscuits, bread, cakes, crackers, oats, pasta, potatoes, rice, sugar, wine, beer, sweets

Hip & Thigh Diet

The principle behind the hip and thigh diet is to drastically reduce fat intake while eating unlimited quantities of vegetables, including potatoes and specified portions of meat and dairy foods. Three meals a day are encouraged, and snacks can be included if the meal quantities are redistributed to accommodate them. A comprehensive exercise programme complements the plan.

Upside:
You do not need to count calories and can eat unlimited quantities of some foods to keep hunger at bay. Weight loss can be impressive, although you are encouraged not just to focus on your weight on the scales, but on inches lost from the important areas such as your thighs.

Downside:
You will need to watch the fat content of your diet to keep within the guidelines. The extremely low fat intake can take some getting used to.

Duration:
Indefinite, if you follow the maintenance diet once sufficient weight is lost.

Checklist:
Restaurants: Possible if you know the foods on the menu and choose the most reduced or low-fat options.
Alcohol: Yes, limited to two drinks per day.
Caffeine: Yes.
Need to buy special foods: No.
Family friendly: A bit too low in fat for children's needs.
OK for vegetarians: Yes, lots of suggestions for veggie meals.

The pros say:
This plan is a little too low in fat compared with UK recommendations. However, the principles are sound in that it encourages high consumption of fruits, vegetables and starchy carbohydrates.

Phase 1 - Fat Attack Fortnight
For the first two weeks you follow the Fat Attack Fortnight, which includes a daily activity challenge to help you get moving and burn extra calories. You eat three main meals a day - breakfast, lunch and dinner plus two power snacks; one mid-morning and one mid-afternoon. You can switch the meals around to suit your daily routine. For these two weeks give alcohol a miss.

Phase 2
From Week 3 you are allowed an extra 300 calories a day. You can do this by adding:
*   One dessert worth 100 calories (max. 5% fat)
*   One treat worth 100 calories - this can be high fat or low fat
*   One alcoholic drink worth 100 calories: e.g. 125ml glass wine; large gin/vodka and slimline mixer; 300ml beer or lager.

Diet rules
*   Each day you should consume 450ml / 3/4pint of skimmed or semi-skimmed milk, which

you can have on breakfast cereals as well as in tea and coffee.

- Drink at least 2 litres of water per day. Low-calorie soft drinks are also unrestricted.
- Lunch usually includes a small salad, which can be saved and eaten as an extra snack or with your main meal in the evening.
- Use fat-free dressings on salads.
- 1 piece of fresh fruit means an orange, apple, pear, or a regular nectarine, peach or 115g fruit such as berries or grapes.

Sample menu

Breakfast
1 Mullerlight Corner Healthy Balance yogurt plus 5 sliced strawberries (V)

Mid-morning Power Snack
1/2 x 35g Rosemary Conley Low Gi Nutrition Bar (eat remaining half on Day 3)

Lunch
1 small granary baguette filled with 50g diced, cooked beetroot, 50g smoked trout fillets plus watercress or rocket leaves, served with 1 blue portion pot/85g virtually fat-free fromage frais mixed with 1 tsp horseradish sauce

Mid-afternoon Power Snack
1 small banana

Dinner
Stir-fry pork with pineapple and rice: Cut 75g lean pork steak into strips and dry-fry in non-stick wok for 2-3 minutes. Add chopped spring onion, 1/2 red onion and 25g mushrooms and cook for further minute, then add 50g fresh beansprouts and a few canned pineapple chunks. In a bowl mix together 2 tbsps pineapple juice, 1 tsp cider vinegar and 2 tsps tomato puree, pour in wok, toss ingredients well and bring to boil. Serve immediately with 1 blue portion pot/55g (uncooked weight) or 1 red portion pot/144g (cooked weight) boiled basmati rice.

Activity challenge
- Walk briskly for 20 minutes
- Do 2 x 8 reps of ab curls:

Lie on back with knees bent, feet hip width apart. Place hands behind head to support neck. Lift head and shoulders off floor, pulling tummy in tight. Lower again slowly, keeping tummy in.

Juice Fast

There are lots of different juice diets around but they are all based on the same idea - that by drinking large amounts of fresh fruit and vegetable juice, you'll detox your system and lose weight at the same time.

Some juice diets are more extreme than others. On one end of the scale, some diets simply encourage you to add juices to your normal diet to boost your vitamin and mineral intake. On the other end of the scale, some people consume nothing but juice for days or even weeks on end. Do not start an extreme juice diet without consulting your doctor first.

How do juice diets work?

Cooking fruit and veg destroys some of its natural goodness but by drinking fresh juice you get maximum goodness from the food.

Investing in a juicer and making your own juices is even better than buying pre-packaged fruit and veg juices as even these have been treated and preservatives added to make them last longer.

Although fruit and veg juices contain natural sugars, they tend to be extremely low in fat so will help you lose weight. There is even some evidence that fresh juice can help fight cancer and other diseases.

People who want to lose weight quickly. People who want to detoxify their systems or wean themselves off drinking too much caffeine or alcohol.

What are the drawbacks?

Detoxing can cause headaches and you may well be hungry on a juice diet if you don't eat other healthy foods as well. If you follow an extreme juice diet, you will probably put back on any weight you've lost pretty quickly.

The best way to start is by buying your own juicer. A cheap blender can be used for softer fruits such as bananas and strawberries but for harder fruits and vegetables, you may need to spend a bit more. You don't have to spend a fortune although there are juicers on the market for up to £500!

Depending on which juice diet you follow, you either add fruit and veg juices to your normal diet or have juice instead of one or more meals a day.

You should aim to drink a variety of fruit and vegetable juices as they all contain different vitamins and minerals. So instead of sticking with just orange or apple, try beetroot, carrot and tomato juice. If you find vegetable juices too sour, add some apple juice to help sweeten them.

Alternatively, if you don't have the time or money to make your own juices, you can buy them from supermarkets or health food shops. Look for freshly-squeezed juices with no added salt or sugar. Decent brands of vegetable juice include V8 and Biotta.

The three phases of the Fasting Diet are:

    Pre-fast diet: This includes three days of high fibre from both raw foods and supplemental fibre. You'll eliminate most sources of fat and protein. A typical day would involve starting the day with a liver/gall bladder tonic called liver flush (three tablespoons of olive oil, one to two cloves of garlic, and the juice of one lemon). You follow the flush with one teaspoon of vegetable fibre, one bowel tablet, and eight to ten ounces of water. You'll repeat this process before lunch and dinner. Breakfast is all fruit and lunch and dinner are all vegetables. Snacks include whole fruit, raw vegetables, raw sunflower seeds, or diluted juices. You should drink at least three quarts of fluid daily.

    The juice diet: For five days you will consume three quarts of vegetable juice (a blend of carrot, celery, and beet juice) each day. You can add some fruit juice, but not citrus or tomato juice, to provide fuel and diversity in taste. You must use an enema since you will not have enough food (and fibre) to relieve yourself naturally. Fear not: the diet provides explicit instructions and pictures to ensure success.

Reintroducing foods: You would ruin the good effects of a long, successful fast by reintroducing complex foods too rapidly. You must gradually add back foods in this order: fruits and non-starchy vegetables, starchy vegetables such as squash and yams, cereals and grains, legumes and fats, and finally nuts and seeds. Introduce new foods or suspect foods one at a time in small amounts to determine if you are sensitive to that particular food.

What are the weight loss expectations for the Fasting Diet?

The Fasting Diet's main purpose is to detoxify and purify the body, rather than to cause weight loss. If you lose weight while on The Fasting Diet and then return to a diet high in processed and refined foods, then you will likely gain back the weight.

Does the Fasting Diet promote exercise?

You should exercise while on The Fasting Diet. You should participate in fun and engaging activities that feel good and are pleasurable enough to maintain on a regular basis.

Does the Fasting Diet recommend supplements?

Supplements are essential. You should add cold-pressed seeds like flax, sunflower, and borage, since the average American diet lacks enough essential fatty acids. You should also take vitamin E and water-soluble vitamins (B vitamins and vitamin C). Drink a smoothie with added flaxseed oil, lecithin granules, protein powder, Nutrizyme, and beta-carotene five days a week for therapeutic purposes and three days a week for health maintenance.

L.A. Shape

The L.A. Shape diet covers all the bases when it comes to weight loss, including advice on exercise, behaviour, and food choices. The use of supplements seems rather intensive, since dieters are supposed to not only eat lots of fruits and veggies but also take supplements containing some of the same phytochemicals found in these fruits and vegetables. The plan also calls for green tea extract and herbals as well as larger amounts of familiar nutrients like vitamin C, vitamin E, and selenium. In addition, to be honest, the information about the relationship between body shape and diet strategies is a little confusing. Heber advises readers with an "apple" shape to take a different diet approach than pear-shaped folks who have extra weight mostly in their hips and thighs. Yet the book tells dieters to use their current weight, not shape, to determine protein levels. And another thing: Some new research suggests dieters might benefit from higher protein levels to promote weight loss, but this approach is still considered preliminary.

Basic principles

The diet downplays simple sugar and fat and focuses on eating protein and building muscle. As a dieter's lean body mass increases, the number of calories he or she burns at rest also increases. One pound of lean body mass, or muscle, burns 14 calories a day, Heber says. He also contends that body shape is important, both for dieting purposes and for overall health. Too much fat around the belly can set the stage for a whole host of health problems, including diabetes and heart disease. Fat around the hips and thighs is less of a health risk.

How the diet works

There are two diet phases. The first phase is a 7-day quick-start plan that calls for dieters to down two "Empowering Shakes," one for breakfast and one for lunch. Supper is a regular meal of "good" carbs, fruits and veggies, and lean meat or fish. By phase two, dieters are increasing food amounts and eating replacements along with seven servings of fruits and veggies and 25 grams of fibre. Supplements including herbals, green tea extract, and added antioxidant nutrients are encouraged. The diet breaks down to 29 percent protein, 20 percent fat, and about 51 percent carbs.

What you can eat

A lot of those "empowering" shakes. Dieters use a blender to whip up different varieties of these homemade meal replacements with fruit, nonfat milk, and protein powder (the recipes are Heber's). For the first week, dieters drink two meal-replacement shakes per day and eat a nutritious supper of 3 to 6 ounces of lean meat or fish, 2 cups of steamed veggies, and 4 cups of salad dressed with vinegar. Dessert is fruit. Eventually, dieters use meal replacements at breakfast only.

"The L.A. shape diet" came out in 2004. It was written by David Heber, professor of medicine and public health, and founding director of the UCLA Centre for Human Nutrition. The diet is based on establishing the right proportion of protein according to individual needs and body shape. Heber suggests an intake of protein almost double the amount recommended at present. He offers Body Mass Index tables to establish what type one is and the corresponding protein intake required.

Permitted Foods

There is no specific list of permitted foods. The direction to follow is high-protein, and low-carb. Heber does not lay particular stress on protein of animal origin, although it is included under good potential protein sources, like previous high-protein diets (such as Atkins or South Beach). Thus the diet might particularly appeal to vegetarians. Heber mentions egg whites, nonfat cottage cheese, soy-based Canadian bacon, tuna, turkey breast, diet products, and meal replacements such as diet shakes consisting of fruit, soy protein and calcium.

The book suggests diet recipes and recommends daily consumption of fruit and vegetables — seven servings a day, each of another color, so as to benefit from each group of fruit and vegetables. This recommendation is based on Heber's theory on fruit and vegetables, which he classifies into seven categories according to their color, each color having particular beneficial properties.

Diet Plan

The 14-Day weight loss plan suggests an individualized approach, based on the dieter's gender, weight and height. For the first week it is recommended that two meals be replaced by diet products (shakes) and that dinner is simple, lean fish or poultry and salad.

Heber gives the key to successful weight-loss, following seven steps:

1. First week — essential to weight loss.
2. Diet personalization — learning what your personal needs are and building a personal diet plan.
3. Applying the personal plan — try to control your eating and develop habits appropriate to your plan.
4. Reinforce your habits — learn to control yourself against external factors. These include stress and stimulus control. Learn coping strategies, and prevent the return to old habits.
5. Inspiration — make an inner approach to integrating the newly achieved practices into your life.
6. Exercise — develop and maintain a personal daily exercise routine.
7. Supplements and herbs — establish your needs for multivitamins, multiminerals and dietary supplements.

Living Low Carb

The objective of all low-carb diets, which date back at least to the early nineteenth century, has always been weight loss. Although plenty of low-fat advocates continue to insist that it's only water that's lost on a low-carb regimen, many patients using it have lost over 100 pounds in short order. Among the many formerly obese, it's pretty well agreed that low-carb is the most effective, most enjoyable, and most successful over the long term of all the various diets. Despite our government's dictate that we load up on carbs to maintain our health, low-carb books have consistently topped the bestseller charts for nearly a decade. Literally millions of people have followed these diets with no reported ill effects so far. Although low-carb diets are still controversial within the health establishment, they have never been vulnerable to charges like the deaths that have been associated with fen-phen or liquid diets. The theoretical argument will continue to rage, and it's extremely unlikely that any definitive studies will be done anytime soon to settle it.

Why do these low-carb diets work so well when almost nothing else does? For a long time the exact mechanisms weren't clearly understood, but when Drs. Michael and Mary Dan Eades (authors of Protein Power) went back to their basic biochemistry texts, they discovered not only the weight-loss mechanism but also the huge number of health benefits that can accrue to many who follow the low-carb path. These include dramatically lowering high blood pressure, levels of the dangerous blood fats called triglycerides, and LDL (bad) cholesterol; controlling diabetes; supplying extra energy throughout the entire day with no up-and-down swings; increasing concentration and focus; enhancing lean body mass with loss of excess body fat; improving immune function; eliminating gout and esophageal reflux; and many other benefits, such as a reversal of inflammatory conditions.

All this happens, the experts in the area now agree, because restricting carbohydrates — sugar and starch in whatever form, from Popsicles to baked potatoes — puts the brakes on insulin, the hormone that's responsible not only for storing fat (and worse, keeping it stored) but also for raising blood pressure, damaging blood vessels, and wreaking other bits of havoc throughout the body for those of us who are genetically predisposed to obesity, diabetes, and heart disease.

Incoming sugars and starches require insulin — the more sugar you consume, the more insulin is needed to process it at the cellular level. After an individual has been on a steady high-sugar diet over a number of years, the insulin receptors on his or her cells may become resistant, in which case even more insulin is required to handle the sugar load. Such a person usually develops insulin resistance, sometimes called Syndrome X or hyperinsulinemia, which usually leads to Type II (adult-onset) diabetes. An insulin-resistant person usually has an increased waist-to-hip ratio, high blood glucose levels, high uric acid, high triglycerides, and low HDL (the good cholesterol). There seems to be a genetic propensity to have problems with insulin. If your family tends to gain weight easily, especially in the abdominal area, you probably have this syndrome, and are therefore at risk for the related health problems (if you don't already have them) unless you change your diet.

The only way to cut back on this outpouring of insulin is by reducing your intake of carbohydrates. Since you always need the same amount of protein, no matter what diet you're on — about 0.5 gram for every pound of your ideal weight — you'll obviously eat more fat on a low-carb diet. (Remember, there are only three food groups to choose from: protein, fat, and carbohydrate.) A number of low-carb diets feature enormous amounts of steak, cheese, butter, and cream, and many anecdotal tales tell of people consuming up to 3,000 calories a day on such a regime and still continuing to lose weight. Other low-carb diets limit the consumption of fats, or vary the ratios of the kinds of fats consumed.

So, do calories not count? They do and they don't. If you don't have insulin problems and have a normal metabolism but simply eat too much, you can go by the standard advice: Cut calories and you will lose weight. But if you do have genetic insulin problems, as you probably do if you're from an overweight family, you may not fare as well on a reduced-calorie diet unless you also cut the carbs very far back. Except for the amazing tales of the 3,000-calorie dieters, though, there's no free lunch on a low-carb diet: If you want to lose a substantial amount of weight, you still need to create a caloric deficit, though perhaps not such a dramatic one as if you weren't concentrating on cutting carbs.

Many people who aren't actually overweight adopt a low-carb diet for health reasons. Some of them are skinny but diabetic; others would prefer to attempt to control their cholesterol or blood pressure without dangerous and expensive medications. The muscular guys you see at the gym eat low-carb to build their lean body mass and minimize fat. Many children with epilepsy have for decades now been given a very successful treatment that involves a no-carb, high-fat diet — not only has their epilepsy been controlled when medication has failed, they've suffered no ill effects from such a drastic regime.

The nutritional establishment's thinking on the subject of dietary fat has begun to change, partly because the low-fat prescription has had fairly unhappy results, such as continuing rampant obesity throughout the population and childhood diabetes increasing by 20 percent in the last decade. Fertility levels have fallen, which may also be a result of our not eating enough fat, and leading researchers such as Dr. Walter Willett of Harvard have started arguing that it's the kind of fat, not the total fat consumed, that makes the difference in weight gain. Willett is comfortable with a diet that's as high as 40 percent fats, as long as those fats are mainly unsaturated.

The fact is, we don't really know very much about human nutrition and metabolism, despite experts' having made claims for "the perfect diet" since the beginning of time. What our species actually evolved to eat, though, is quite like the low-carb diet: protein and fat from small animals and sea creatures and birds, small amounts of carbohydrate from plants and berries and seeds and nuts, and the occasional feast on a major animal. Dairy products are quite recent additions to the human diet, as are agricultural products, which we've had for only 10,000 years — a minuscule amount of time, from an evolutionary standpoint. Many of us may simply not have adapted biologically to this relatively "new" diet, which may be one reason we feel so good and flourish so well on a low-carb plan.

Needless to say, there are many theories within the low-carb camp, and many different low-carb regimens. If you're seriously thinking about eating this way for the rest of your life — as you should be if you have the insulin problem — you ought to take a look at all of them and choose the one that seems best suited to you.

What It Is

Since low-carbohydrate dieting has taken America by storm, it was only natural that cookbooks would follow. First came *The Low-Carb Cookbook,* succeeded by *Living Low-Carb,* both by Fran McCullough, an avowed foodie and award-winning cookbook editor. Struggling to keep her own weight down, McCullough was led to a low-carb diet, which suited her to a T. In her quest for meal-time pleasure without plumpness, she put together a collection of more than 250 recipes for the 1997 *The Low-Carb Cookbook.* The book was an instant success and best seller. *Living Low-Carb* followed in 2000, which contains more explanation and adds 175 recipes.

McCullough's latest book explains the differences between the most stringent low-carb diet plans and the more liberal ones that she favours. She then outlines how to adapt the latter group of diets to fit a pleasure-eater's perspective. Rather than a "diet" book, *Living Low-Carb* is more of a lifestyle and self-help guide with recipes for everything from home fries to Moroccan-styled chicken to what she calls Intense Chocolate Cake.

McCullough dismisses the raft of objections to the low-carb diet by the nutritional establishment, but she does note that for some people this type of routine is not ideal. She discusses the particular needs of diabetics, those with low-thyroid function (her own condition), and includes caveats for those pregnant or nursing. *Living Low-Carb* is full of motivational suggestions, as well as practical ones for stocking the pantry, eating on the road, in restaurants, and at the homes of friends, and finally how to deal with a dieter's bete noir, the sweet tooth.

She encourages exercise, not because it will make you lose fat, but because it's good for you, and she gives you more than a dozen reasons why you should.

How It Works

McCullough gives you lots of choices, because neither *Living Low-Carb* nor *The Low-Carb Cookbook* is a diet book as such. The recipes are for everything from canapes to desserts. However, she does present a basic plan for low-carb eating:

- Have protein at every meal -- about one-half gram of protein for every pound of your ideal weight, typically somewhere between 60 to 85 grams unless you're very large or very small.
- For weight loss, keep the carbs low, anywhere from zero to 30 grams daily.
- Choose whole foods, organic if possible, and raw, ideally. The more fibre, the better.
- Avoid nearly everything white -- potatoes, rice, bread, flour, sugar, popcorn. Of course, this doesn't include cauliflower, turnips or giant white radishes.
- Eat fruit at breakfast, particularly low-carb fruits, such as berries, melon, peaches, kiwi. Half a banana is all you get.
- Although you are allowed cream and butter, save it for treats, and cut down on them if you are trying to lose weight. Choose cold-pressed olive and nut oils, and avoid processed oils, partially hydrogenated fats and margarine.
- Eat dinner early and make it minimal.

Now, what about the recipes? All are low-carb with the exception of several moderately higher-carb dessert recipes. McCullough points out that the carbohydrate counts she gives will not be the same as those in standard books, because the fibre count has been subtracted from the total carb count. What does that mean? The fibre component, she says, is not metabolically active and does not raise blood sugar levels, which allows you to have more carbs if they are in the form of fibre. Appetizers include roasted almonds, grilled Parmesan chunks and stuffed mushrooms; main courses include pork tenderloin, several ways of preparing salmon and something called A Lot Like Lasagna, made with zucchini, spinach, Italian sausage and ricotta; desserts run from Rummy Pumpkin Mousse to Capri Chocolate Almond Torte.

Sample Meals

Green Eggs and Ham

Lighter than bacon and eggs or eggs with cheese, this zesty combination is particularly appealing on a summer morning–or for a light supper.

SERVES 2
6 large eggs
Salt and pepper to taste
Dash of water
Dash of hot pepper sauce (optional)
2 tablespoons butter
2 scallions, minced, including the firm green part
1 cup chopped fresh cilantro
2 tablespoons chopped fresh dill
2 ounces ham, diced

Whisk the eggs in a bowl, adding the salt and pepper, water, and hot pepper sauce and mixing well. Melt the butter in a skillet and when it's foaming, add the scallions. Sauté a couple of minutes. Pour the seasoned eggs into the skillet and scatter the cilantro and dill on top. With a spatula, turn back the edges of the eggs and let the uncooked egg on top take their place. Begin to gently scramble them and scatter the diced ham on top.

Cook the eggs to the degree of wetness you like and serve.

Per Serving:
Carbohydrate: 3.4g plus 1.3g fibre
Protein: 26.2g
Fat: 29.2g

Tuna Salad with Beans and Broccoli

On a hot night–or just a busy one when there's no time to cook– this salad can be dinner in moments. I used to make a salad like this one with garbanzo beans, which you could also use, but your carb debt would go way up. You'll find these black soybeans are a tasty alternative.

SERVES 6

6 1/2-ounce can tuna packed in olive oil, drained
15-ounce can Eden black soybeans, rinsed under running water
1 cup broccoli florets, steamed 5 minutes or microwaved just until tender
2 scallions, chopped, including the firm part of the green
Half a red bell pepper, cored, seeded, and diced
Handful of fresh basil, chopped
Handful of fresh parsley, chopped
2 tablespoons olive oil
2 teaspoons red wine vinegar
1 garlic clove
Salt and pepper

Mix the tuna, soybeans, broccoli, scallions, red pepper, basil, and parsley together in a serving bowl.

In a small bowl, mix the oil and vinegar. Spear the garlic clove on a fork and use the fork to whisk the oil and vinegar together until they begin to emulsify. Add salt and pepper to taste. Whisk again with the garlic clove and pour over the salad, tossing well to combine.

Per Serving:
Carbohydrate: 5g plus 5.6g fibre
Protein: 21.8g
Fat: 13.5g

Lime Mousse

This tart, airy, creamy dessert is perfect after Mexican or Indian meals. You can also freeze it in an ice cream maker for a summer sorbet. And it couldn't be easier to make, especially if you have a rasp.

When key limes are in season in early spring, or when you see the little Mexican limes in the market, snap them up and make this marvellous mousse. It's so good, in fact, that I can happily eat the entire thing by myself, so be warned.

SERVES 4

1/4 cup warm water
1 (1/4-ounce) envelope unflavoured powdered gelatin
I tablespoon grated lime zest
1/2 cup fresh lime juice, strained (about 4 limes or 18 key limes)
1/3 cup Splenda low-calorie sweetener; or more to taste

1 cup sour cream

3 egg whites, at room temperature

Put the warm water in a glass bowl and sprinkle the gelatin over it. Let sit 5 minutes, then microwave on high 20 seconds, or until dissolved. Stir to be sure no lumps remain; if they do, microwave until they disappear.

In a 4-cup souffle dish, combine the gelatin, the lime zest, and juice and stir well. Add the Splenda and the sour cream and stir again.

Beat the egg whites just until you have soft peaks, adding a few drops of lime juice from one of the squeezed limes to stabilize the whites. Fold the egg whites into the lime mixture.

Cover the dish with plastic wrap and refrigerate 4 hours before serving.

Per Serving:

Carbohydrate: 5.4g plus 0.2g fibre

Protein: 6.1g

Fat: 12.1g

Low Fat

The logic of these diets is that, because fat contains more calories than carbohydrates or protein, limiting the fat in our diet is a simple way to promote weight loss.

All types of added fats, such as butter, margarine, mayonnaise, sour cream and salad dressings, are reduced or eliminated. Foods high in fat, such as fried foods, snack foods, cheeses and red meat, should be replaced with lower-fat versions or eaten in smaller portions. Most low-fat diets call for an increase of carbohydrate intake in the form of pasta, breads and potatoes.

A high-fat diet has been associated with numerous health conditions, from obesity to heart disease and even some types of cancer. The plan encourages the use of foods naturally low in fat, such as fruits and vegetables, which also contain healthy amounts of essential nutrients .

Upside of Low Fat Diets
- Foods that are low in fat - for example, vegetables, whole grains, fruit - are generally healthy.
- Many high fat foods are also high in sugar, which is bad for you and can lead to weight gain. Cutting down on cookies and ice cream is never a bad thing!
- A low-fat diet has been shown to reduce the risk of many health conditions, including high cholesterol, heart disease and obesity.

Downside of Low Fat Diets
- Not all foods that are low in fat are also low in calories. For example, bread and pasta are both fairly low in fat but can pile on the calorie intake if eaten to excess.
- There has been an explosion of foods that are reduced in fat yet contain lots of sugar: snack bars, cookies, cakes, candies, ice cream and so on. Those foods do not promote a healthy diet, even if they are low in fat.
- Low-fat diets assume that all fat is created equal, which researchers now know is not the case. Monounsaturated fats, the type found in olive oil and certain oily fish, have been found to be essential to a healthy body and mind.
- Some vitamins (e.g., vitamins A, E and K) are found predominantly in fatty foods. People who eat a low-fat diet normally are advised to take vitamin supplements.
- Fat makes food taste better - it's sad but true. Therefore, if you try to eliminate fat from your diet, you end up with boring, bland meals, making it less likely that you'll stick to the diet.

Sample Low Fat Diet Menu

A traditional low fat diet consists mainly of foods that are low in fat and high in fibre. Some people may wish to add foods that contain monounsaturated fats, such as avocado and nuts:

Breakfast:
- Oatmeal made with skim milk, topped with blueberries
- Cup of herbal tea

Lunch:
- Ginger carrot soup with whole-wheat bread
- Pear, apple and cranberry fruit salad

Dinner:
- Mediterranean chicken over whole-wheat spaghetti
- Roasted vegetables
- Small glass of red wine
- Sliced melon with cherries

Snacks:
- Celery sticks or broccoli and low-fat ranch dressing
- Low-fat cottage cheese (or fat-free yogurt) with fresh fruit

On the whole, the foods that are encouraged on low-fat diets are generally healthy, and cutting down on fat is a fairly efficient way to lose weight. However, it's important to remember that fat isn't the only source of calories in your diet, and many foods that are touted as "low fat" may be high in calories.

Also, over the last 10 years, there has been increasing evidence to show that some fats may actually be good for us and should be included in our diets. If you're thinking of taking on a low-fat diet, make sure you're getting rid of saturated fats and trans fats while taking in enough monounsaturated fats.

Mayo Clinic Diet

Although the New Mayo Clinic Diet has spread like wilfdfire and is responsible for millions of pounds in weight loss, the Mayo Clinic reports it, "did not originate at Mayo Clinic," nor is it, "approved by Mayo Clinic."

BREAKFAST:
    1/2 grapefruit or 8oz unsweetened juice.
    2 Eggs any style
    2 Slices of bacon
    Black coffee or tea, no sugar

LUNCH:
    1/2 grapefruit or 8oz unsweetened juice.
    Salad and or raw veggies (any dressing, {not low fat or fat free})
    Meat (Cooked any way)

DINNER:
    1/2 grapefruit or 8oz unsweetened juice.
    Meat (cooked any way) Vegetables (any green or red, may be cooked in butter or Seasoning or a salad as above) Black coffee or tea, no sugar

BEDTIME:
    (opt) 8oz Tomato juice or skim milk

INSTRUCTIONS:
    1. At any meal you may eat until you are full, and you can not eat anymore. You must eat the minimum listed at each meal.
    2. Do not eliminate anything from the diet, especially don't skip the bacon at breakfast or omit salads. It is the combination of foods that burn the fat.
    3. The grapefruit is important because it acts as a catalyst that starts the burning process.
    4. Cut down on coffee, it affects the insulin balance that hinders the burning process. Try to limit to one cup each meal.
    5. Don't eat between meals, if you eat the combination of food suggested, you will not get hungry.
    6. The diet may eliminate sugars and starches. Fat does not form fat, it helps burn it, so you can fry food in butter and use butter generously on vegetables.
    7. Do not eat desserts, breads and white vegetables of sweet potatoes. You may double or triple helpings of meat, salads or vegetables. Eat till you are stuffed. The more you eat the more weight you will lose.
    8. There may be no weight loss in the first 4 days, but you may lose 5 pounds on the 5th day. You may lose 1 and 1/2 pounds every two days until you reach your goal.
    9. DRINK EIGHT 8oz GLASSES OF WATER EVERY DAY. 1/2 GALLON.
THIS DIET IS SAID TO BEEN GIVEN TO HEART PATIENTS NEEDING TO LOSE WEIGHT FAST FOR BY-PASS SURGERY.
ALL SOFT DRINKS NEED TO BE DIET AND CAFFEINE FREE.
YOU MAY NOT HAVE: White onions, potatoes, celery, peas, cereal, carrots, corn, starchy vegetables, bread, noodles, rice, potato chips, pretzels or fruit or diet dressing.

YOU MAY HAVE: Red onions, bell peppers, radishes, broccoli, cucumbers, green onions, leaf spinach, cabbage, tomatoes, green beans, lettuce, chilli (no beans) mayonnaise, any cheese, hot dogs, coleslaw, regular salad dressing, green vegetables, 1tsp nuts, dill or bread and butter pickles.

IMPORTANT
STAY ON DIET 12 DAYS AND STOP FOR 2 DAYS
Works out great to start on a Monday because you will have every other weekend off of the diet.

Nutrisystem

NutriSystem started out as a weight loss centre-based diet program, like Weight Watchers and Jenny Craig, but has now repositioned itself as an online weight-management program. The core of the plan relies on NutriSystem foods used as entrees for breakfast, lunch and dinner as well as snacks. You don't have to buy their pre-packaged foods to participate in the program, but the NutriSystem meals revolve around the NuCrusine foods, making it difficult to follow the plan without buying the products. The entrees are also supplemented with fruits, vegetables, and skim milk.

All the meals and snacks fit into an easy-to-follow meal plan that stresses proper portions and eating six times a day to fuel your metabolism and keep you from feeling hungry. The meals are carefully calorie controlled so the dieter does not need to count calories in order to lose weight.

How Nutrisystem Diet Works

The NutriSystem Diet is divided into two phases: weight loss, followed by weight maintenance. In the first phase, dieters eat NutriSystem pre-packaged foods seven days a week and supplement these meals with fresh fruits, vegetables, and skim milk. The time spent on the reduced caloric diet depends on individual goal weights. The weight-maintenance program generally lasts up to one year, during which dieters eat NutriSystem foods two days a week and regular foods the other five days of the week.

There are more than 100 different pre-packaged, shelf-stable, microwaveable NuCuisine entrees and snacks to choose from, including entrees that range from Tex-Mex Rice and Beans to Spicy Oriental Noodles with vegetables and peanuts, to old standbys like macaroni and cheese. Dieters can make their own menus from the pre-packaged foods, or they can choose from diet meal packages suited to different tastes, such as Active Lifestyle, All-American, Healthy Lifestyles, International Light and Lean, and Traditional Favourites.

Advantages of the Nutrisystem Diet
- The NutriSystem Diet emphasizes the role of regular exercise, provides a weekly newsletter and chat rooms, and includes a weekly one-on-one email chat with a personal counsellor to help you stay on track.
- The meal plan is based on low-fat food choices from the Food Guide Pyramid and recommends a balanced diet that includes all types of foods.

Disadvantages of the Nutrisystem Diet
- The NutriSystem NuCuisine foods cost about $50 a week, so you need to examine your budget before signing on to the program.
- This plan works well if you're single or eat alone; however, if you have a family to cook for you'll either need to buy enough NutriSystem meals for everyone or prepare two separate meals.

Dieticians Comments About Nutrisystem Diet

Overall, the NutriSystem Diet is a nutritionally sound, reduced-calorie diet. The diet was developed in accordance with weight-loss recommendations from the American Dietetic Association and the National Institutes of Health. This program is perfect for someone who likes structure and pre-packaged convenience foods, and doesn't like to cook. However, anyone who craves the fresh taste of pan sautéed fish, roasted chicken, or a sizzling steak right off the grill isn't going to be won over by the taste of freeze-dried scrambled eggs.

Like the Jenny Craig Diet plan and other similar programs that offer preplanned menus with packaged foods, nutritionists have reservations with the NutriSystem Diet. Dieters should be prepared to learn how to maintain weight loss by making the right food and cooking choices once the diet program is over.

Picture Perfect

You can develop the skills to make healthier eating choices with Dr. Howard Shapiro's Guide to Picture Perfect Weight Loss. He's developed a program around Food Awareness Training. Dr. Shapiro says it's the choices you make that have the most impact and will help you find ways to incorporate more filling, delicious foods and snacks into your diet without loading up on calories.

The Picture Perfect Guide dieters follow photos to gain perspective on their eating habits. Dr. Shapiro compares several lean servings of calorie-packed foods against bigger servings of low-calorie foods to show you how easy the choices can be. For instance, for 1,360 calories you could indulge in an ice cream sundae with the works- chocolate sauce, nuts and whipped cream. Or, for 1,360 calories you could have four frozen yogurt sundaes with chocolate sauce and whipped cream (or just enjoy one sundae for 1/4 of the calories). While you wouldn't sit down to eat four sundaes, the point is that you can treat yourself to the sweet things you love, without packing on all the unnecessary calories.

Picture Perfect Weight Loss dieters will be able to maintain their ability to make better eating choices after the 30-day plan is completed because Dr. Shapiro suggests the photos will serve as a constant reminder of the healthy choices that are so easy to make.

FOOD & RECIPE
You're given alternatives that may be shocking. You can lose 50 percent of your breakfast calories by replacing an on-the-go toaster pastry with toaster waffles, light syrup and fresh blueberries. For dinner, skip greasy chicken quesadillas and try shrimp with salsa, rice, beans and baby squash.

EXERCISE
Dr. Shapiro's plan centres on food choices, not exercise.

EXPENSE
Cost of the book Dr. Shapiro's Picture Perfect Weight Loss: The Visual Program for Permanent Weight Loss.

PRO
Dr. Shapiro's approach is very effective, in that it he reveals the amazing difference in food calorie content.

CON
Is there a downside to a plan created by the same person who helped the New York City Police Department and Fire Departments lose weight?
This is the true "see food" diet. The Picture Perfect diet shows you pictures of different foods so that you can learn to make intelligent eating choices. Filled with color photography, the book for this diet also provides nutritional tips to help you understand how to get the most out of your daily food selections. Many pages offer choices between two full-page photographs. On one side, for instance, is the picture of plain dry bagel (400 calories). On the other, is a photo of an English muffin with jam (170 calories). The idea of the Picture Perfect Diet is that you can become educated about the implications of what you eat. Then, this comprehension of the real calories in

your selections will help you make wise eating choices. You don't weigh or measure foods, or count every calorie.

What makes The Picture Perfect Diet a different weight loss program?
No gimmicks, no crazy rules, no supplements. You use realistic images of foods (more than 115 in all) that you currently eat. You can compare the images and nutritional information with foods you might want to eat instead. If you are a visual learner, this diet is for you.

What is The Picture Perfect Diet Weight Loss Program?
This program encourages you to open your eyes and pay attention to what you are eating. Its goal is to help you recognize healthier food options that you would enjoy and find satisfying. The diet's "Fat Awareness Training" includes nutrition education and guidelines to create meals without complex plans or recipes. You'll also acquire nutrition savvy through visual imagery, label reading, and shopping tips.

The Picture Perfect Diet plan provides four basic eating profiles. You must decide which category fits you best. The choices include: the workaholic who is too busy to eat during the day; the business traveller who eats and drinks as part of the job; the parent at home with the kids; and the student or shift worker who keeps unusual hours and is always on the run. The Picture Perfect Diet program tracks the eating behaviours and food diaries of these profiles, points out the factors affecting each group's poor eating, and supplies options for better food choices tailored to each group's specific needs and schedules.

Most important are the pictorial food examples. You'll be able to look at common meals and snacks, vegetarian options, traditional holiday foods, international cuisines, and familiar restaurant fare. The idea is to illustrate the amount of calories in different food options. After all, would you rather have one fat-free cookie or an entire cantaloupe?

Some examples of the Picture Perfect Diet include:
- Instead of a Frosted Blueberry Pop Tarts (420 calories), choose two low-fat waffles, one tablespoon light syrup, and blueberries (250 calories).
- Instead of 2 2/3 ounces of mixed nuts (400 calories), choose ten cups of popcorn (also 400 calories) - or better yet, have 3 cups and save the calories.
- One raspberry tart (440 calories) is equal to eight cups of raspberries with whipped topping.
- Some pictures help to visualize the amount of fat in foods by depicting fat content with pats of butter: a cup of premium ice cream is equal to ten pats of butter.

Try to avoid eating processed fat-free foods, meats, dairy, and poultry on the Picture Perfect Diet. It's also good to avoid alcohol because its consumption may interfere with thoughtful food choices. You'll also get tips on grocery shopping, label reading, and ordering at restaurants. An "Anytime List" suggests snacks, beverages, condiments, and candy that you should always have available for quick cooking and snacking. You won't get any recipes, but you will find tips on cooking methods and nutrition lessons. This new knowledge will help you understand why one raisin scone has as many calories as 14 slices of raisin bread.

What are the weight loss expectations?
The Picture Perfect Diet contains no specific weight loss promises because there are numerous factors that influence food choices, especially calorie reduction and exercise. More time on the diet will hopefully enhance your skills and lead to continual and maintained weight loss.

Is exercise promoted?

Exercise is a very important component to the Picture Perfect Diet. If you're serious about losing weight, you should be exercising. Find ways to increase exercise during daily activities such as housework and shopping trips. Get moving and don't wait just for designated exercise times. One recommendation that you may particularly enjoy is that it's good to visit lavish health spas. Spas do promote exercise and often offer many healthy food choices as part of their menus. This can be very therapeutic if it falls within your budget.

Are supplements recommended?

Do not take supplements, according to the Picture Perfect Diet. There is not enough scientific research to support their safe and/or effective use. There is no federal regulation to protect you when purchasing these products.

CONCLUSION

While Dr. Shapiro's Guide is calorie-driven, dieters are encouraged to not count their calories and instead make lower calorie choices. He suggests that counting calories is where dieters find frustration when trying to lose weight. Dr. Shapiro also steers clear of other common dieting fodder - like meal times, portion sizes and restricted foods. The Picture Perfect plan relies on dieters' minds by using compelling images to motivate.

Dr Phil

This diet by TV psychologist Dr. Phil McGraw promises to free you from your weight loss struggles with seven strategies: Believe you'll succeed, don't look to food to solve your emotional pain, free your environment from trigger foods and reminders to eat, establish a new relationship with food, choose foods that produce and reinforce lasting weight loss, prioritize exercise, and surround yourself with people who support your efforts.

It's no surprise, of course, that the bulk of the psychologist's approach focuses on changing the way you think about yourself, dieting, food and your health. To accomplish that, there are various quizzes throughout the book to determine your current thought and behavioural patterns to understand how they contribute to your weight. Once you've figured out where you stand, Dr. Phil leads you through the steps you need to take to implement changes.

But it's not just all psychology; physical activity and healthier eating are also part of the plan. Dr. Phil separates food into two categories: high-response, high-yield foods versus low-response, low-yield foods. Essentially, this means choosing low-calorie, nutrient-dense foods over high-calorie, low-nutrient foods. He provides serving recommendations and food lists to help you create the three daily meals and two snacks he recommends.
There are seven rules in the book, which are as follows

1) Own Your Reactions: Dr Phil says you can choose your reaction, in any situation. For instance if you are rejected from an interview, don't eat a big packet of chips or don't order for a big hamburger as you feel more like a loser. Don't get upset and rather try to be positive, as that way you will surely get the next job. Positive thinking such as considering the job which you got rejected was not for you would be better.

2) Not only react to the problem but solve the problems: Dr. Phil says always think about the solution but not the reaction. Winning or worrying about the money won't make you lose weight

3) Slow down your thinking: Dr. Phil says that you have to decelerate the process of gaining weight. Slowly think and listen what your thoughts say and then try to pen it down.

4) Challenge yourself: The program of Dr. Phil also suggests you to change your mind. You have to change your beliefs and attitude. By following that only you can get the result, you will be free from negative thinking. You must accept the fact that only you are the reason for getting upset and only you can do something about it.

5) Seek closure: Dr. Phil says do not get angry or damage anything or do not hate any one or take vengeance on any one, which only leads you to many problems. You cannot change other people, but at least you can change the way you respond to them. Never take revenge.

6) Forgive: forgiving is a little tough but it is not an impossible task. As per Dr. Phil's book forgiveness should be a part of your life. It makes you free from anger or emotional upsets which tend to make you eat more food.

7) Manage without food: Dr. Phil's book suggests you to do yoga, meditation and exercise. He also says you could do with listening to music as it will give you the natural motivation to become thin.

If you follow the rules and tips of Dr.Phils you will surely get a good result.

Sample menu

BREAKFAST
Whole-wheat waffles with strawberries and 1% or fat-free milk

LUNCH
Mediterranean salmon salad in pita pocket and fruit

DINNER
Chicken kabobs, brown rice, salad and fruit

SNACKS
1. Shape Up! Chocolate Toffee Crunch Bar
2. Fruit cocktail with graham crackers

Pritikin

The Pritikin Diet was developed by Nathan Pritikin, founder of the Pritikin Longevity Centre in California, as an attempt to markedly reduce the risk of heart disease. Although not principally a weight loss diet, many people who follow the Pritikin Diet tend to lose weight.
The Pritikin Diet is a low-fat, high-carbohydrate eating plan. It focuses on complex carbohydrates, fresh fruits, and vegetables eaten raw or cooked. It is high in fibre, low in cholesterol, and extremely low in saturated fat and total fat, containing less than 10% of total daily calories from fat. The consumption of seafood, rich in omega-3 fatty acids, is encouraged, followed by skinless chicken, and lean red meat.

How Pritikin Diet Works
While the Pritikin Diet doesn't have you counting calories, it does require calculating the average caloric density of each meal, which is done by combining the different caloric food groups. The basic idea is to fill up on low-caloric and medium-caloric density foods that have relatively few calories per pound, such as apples and oatmeal with only occasional forays into high-caloric density foods. The higher the caloric density of any given food, the more likely it is to cause weight gain. Corn, for instance, starts out at a somewhat reasonable 490 calories per pound, but chocolate chip cookies skyrocket to 2,140 calories per pound.
The Pritikin Diet provides menu examples and general dietary suggestions that emphasize eating whole, unprocessed foods like fruits, vegetables, and low-fat carbohydrate foods. This emphasis on complex carbohydrates makes it high in vitamins, minerals, and fibre, and low in sodium. In short, it encompasses a very healthy range of foods and generous portions, which should fill you up without any danger of weight gain.

Advantages of Pritikin Diet
- The Pritikin Diet is good for those folks with a family history of heart disease.
- It encourages eating balanced meals that include high-fibre fruits, vegetables, beans, and grains.

Disadvantages of Pritikin Diet
- The Pritikin Diet is difficult for many people because they have to give up animal products and dairy products.
- Most dieters may have a difficult time sticking to this diet with its low daily intake of fat at 10%.

Dieticians Comments About Pritikin Diet
There seems to be little dispute that you will lose weight with this diet. However, the extremely low fat content of this diet (10% of total calories) will make those following it often feel hungry resulting in the likelihood the weight will return after one stops strictly adhering to the diet. Another problem is that the fat content being so low may be harmful to our health. Because dietary fat is so severely restricted, Pritikin dieters may not be able to consume a sufficient amount of the healthy fats, especially the omega-3 fats. In addition, absorption of the fat-soluble vitamins (A, D, E, and K) may be impaired with such low intakes of dietary fat.

Foods Allowed:
Staples of the Pritikin program: fruits, vegetables, whole grains, beans, peas and potatoes. Modest amounts of nonfat dairy foods, fish, poultry and very lean red meats are allowed.

Foods Restricted:
Most types of processed foods, high fat foods, caffeine, sugar, sweets, alcohol and salt.

Sample Menu:

Breakfast:
1/2 cup oatmeal with 1.5 tablespoon jam
1 cup nonfat fruit yogurt
1 cup nonfat milk
1 cup chickory coffee

Morning Snack:
1/2 medium whole wheat bagel
1/2 medium cantelope

Lunch:
1 medium baked potato with 1/2 cup marinara sauce
1.5 cups mixed salad greens
3/4 cup fresh fruit
1 whole wheat roll

Afternoon Snack:
1/2 cup raw broccoli
1/2 cup cauliflower
2 tablespoons nonfat ranch dressing

Dinner:
1 serving chicken curry
1 cup asparagus
3 cups mixed salad greens
1/2 cup wild rice
1/2 cup skim milk
1 tablespoon chutney

Radiant Health Diet

This diet works on the principle that the more carbs you eat the more you'll want, and too many carbs will sabotage your chances of permanent weight loss. The plan initially treats nutritional deficiencies that cause these cravings and slowly gets you used to eating less carbohydrates. The result is that you store less fat and burn the fat you do have more easily. Carbohydrates are limited to under 70g a day and fruits and vegetables are kept to small portions. You are encouraged to make meats, eggs and cheese the mainstays of your diet. In addition, you need a daily supplement containing essential fatty acids, multiple minerals, essiac and cat's claw to treat deficiencies and detoxify the body.

upside
- Some people enjoy eating lots of meat, eggs and cheese which are usually restricted in traditional low-fat diet plans.
- Often people do notice a drop in their cravings for carbs when they eat a high-protein, high-fat diet, and there are plenty of recipes in this plan to choose from.
- Many people are put off by high-fibre diets because they involve eating lots of fruit and vegetables.
- This diet claims you'll have more energy, less bloating, reduced water retention and improved bowel function within two to three weeks and you will achieve permanent weight loss.

downside
- Cutting down on fruit and veg means you're missing out on important antioxidant nutrients such as vitamin C and other phytochemicals. Too much fat can also lead to heart problems.
- Restricting carbohydrates means the body has to rely primarily on protein (muscle) and fat for its energy reserves. When fat and protein are metabolised, by-products called ketones are produced which can be dangerous for people with diabetes, kidney problems and other medical conditions.
- There is an enormous amount of cooking involved and you're likely to need to cook at least two meals a day.
- Because protein-rich sources are the mainstay of the diet, this plan will be expensive to follow. You also need to buy either the Radiant Health Basic Essence EFA supplement or make up your own cocktail containing EFA, multiple minerals, and supplements essaic and cat's claw.

duration
Two to three weeks.

checklist
Restaurants: You'll need to limit pasta, potatoes, bread, rice, fruit and vegetables.
Alcohol In moderation.
OK for vegetarians: No.
Family friendly: Could be difficult if you have children who enjoy eating bread, potatoes and pasta.
Need to buy special foods: No, but you'll need to buy supplements.
Caffeine: Tea and coffee allowed.

the pros says
It's difficult to eat large amounts of foods on a high-protein, low-carbohydrate diet and this is why you may lose weight initially. Permanent weight loss will be difficult to sustain.

Slim Fast

On the Slim·Fast Optima™ Diet, you can Mix and Match your favourite foods in a variety of ways to create Sensible Meals. Fit the foods you like into Slim·Fast Meal combinations and then pick and choose recipes and familiar favourites to create Sensible Meals. Don't forget you can snack between meals too!

On the Slim·Fast Optima™ Diet, you can Mix and Match your favourite foods in a variety of ways to create Sensible Meals. The Optima™ Sensible Meal should contain approximately 500 calories. But how do you know what a 500 calorie meal looks like?

We'll show you

The Perfect Portions Guideline below is a great visual for you to keep in mind-whether you're preparing food at home or dining out. Always fill 1/2 of your plate with veggies, 1/4 with lean protein (such as chicken without the skin, turkey, fish or lean beef), 1/4 with starch, and enjoy a salad on the side and fruit for dessert. It's that easy!

Protein Choices:
lean beef, pork, poultry, fish, eggs, low-fat cheese, tofu & soy meat products

Vegetable Choices:
green beans, carrots, cauliflower, cabbage, eggplant, spinach, peas, broccoli, asparagus, peppers, mushrooms, squash (all types)

Starch Choices:
potatoes, corn, pasta/noodles, rice, whole wheat bread

Slim·Fast Meal Combinations
The Slim·Fast Meal Combination is a Slim·Fast Meal plus other healthy food choices, such as a half sandwich, yogurt with fruit, or even a Grilled Chicken Caesar Salad with light dressing. You can create your own Slim·Fast Meal Combinations by adding 150 calories of your favourite foods to a Slim·Fast Meal.

Breakfast Combinations
Enjoy a Slim·Fast Meal Option with one of the following:
- Small size café latte made with skim milk
- Whole grain English muffin & 2 teaspoons of light margarine (no trans/sat fat)
- 2 slices 'light' wheat bread & 2 teaspoons of light margarine (no trans/sat fat)
- 1 slice frozen French toast with 1 Tablespoon syrup
- 1 whole wheat pita with 2 tsp sugar-free all-fruit spread
- 1 apple with 1 Tablespoon of reduced fat peanut butter
- 1 packet of instant oatmeal
- 3/4 cup bran flakes with 1/2 cup skim milk
- 1 small fat-free yogurt with 1/4 cup high fibre cereal or low-fat granola
- 1 small fat-free yogurt with 1 cup of berries
- 1 cup of low-fat (1%) cottage cheese
- 1/2 cup of low-fat cottage cheese with 15 grapes
- 1 low-fat whole grain waffle with 2 teaspoons of light margarine
- 4 egg whites on 2 slices of light wheat bread

Lunch/Dinner Combinations

Enjoy a Slim·Fast Meal Option with one of the following:

- 2 ounces of sliced turkey on light wheat bread with mustard
- 1 cup green salad with 2 oz grilled chicken and fat-free dressing
- 1 cup low fat creamy tomato soup (or other low-fat soup)
- Light wheat bread with 2 ounces of lean ham & mustard
- 1/2 roasted chicken breast or two chicken drumsticks without the skin
- 1/2 roast beef sandwich (2 oz roast beef, 1 slice whole wheat bread, 1 tablespoon horseradish, lettuce, tomato)
- 2 ounces of roasted turkey over 1 cup of salad greens with fat-free dressing
- 1 baked potato with 2 tbsp fat free sour cream
- 1 small fat-free yogurt mixed with 1/4 cup high fibre cereal
- 1 cup of baby carrots and 3 tablespoons of hummus
- 12 almonds or other nuts
- 1 cup of salad greens, mixed vegetables, 5 olives and 2 oz of tuna
- 2 slices light wheat bread, 1 Tbsp reduced-fat peanut butter, 1 Tbsp of sugar-free all-fruit spread

Sample Day Diet 1

Breakfast

Slim·Fast Optima Tropical Orange Smoothie
&
3/4 Cup Bran Flakes with 1/2 cup skim milk

Snack

Slim·Fast Optima Blueberry Muffin Bar
&
1 orange

Lunch

2 cups Garden Salad with 2 Tbsp fat-free dressing
1 mini snack box (1/2 oz) raisins
&
Slim·Fast Optima Strawberry Cheesecake Meal Bar

Snack

1 apple
&
1 cup of baby carrots with 2 tbsp fat-free ranch dressing

Dinner

Chicken Veggies Grill: 4 oz. Grilled chicken breast (no skin)
1 small baked potato with 2 Tbsp fat-free sour cream
1 cup steamed broccoli with
1 Tbsp Parmesan cheese
&

1 cup melon

Snack
Slim·Fast Optima Peanut Butter Crunch Snack Bar

Sample Day Diet 2

Breakfast
Slim·Fast Optima Cappuccino Shake
&
1 slice frozen French toast with 1 Tbsp light syrup

Snack
1 cup grapes

Lunch
Slim·Fast Optima French Vanilla Shake
&
1/2 roast beef sandwich
(2 oz. Roast beef, 1 slice whole wheat bread, 1 tbsp horseradish, lettuce, tomato)

Snack
1 piece of part skim mozzarella string cheese
&
1 apple

Dinner
Spaghetti and meatballs:
1 cup spaghetti noodles (cooked)
3 oz. Lean ground beef (shaped into three 1 oz. Meatballs, add seasoning to preference)
1/2 cup marinara spaghetti sauce
2 cups garden salad with 2 tbsp fat-free Italian dressing
&
1 cup strawberries

Snack
One slice low fat pound cake

South Beach Diet

Most people are sick of trying new diets for one reason – they do not work! What makes the South Beach Diet different is that it teaches a way of life where you rely on the right carbohydrates and fats. This new way of eating allows you to live contently without eating the bad carbohydrates and fats. In contrast, when a person eats bad carbohydrates and fats they feel hungrier, causing them to eat more, which causes weight gain. In exchange for eating right, you become healthier and can enjoy an 8 to 13 pound weight loss in just two weeks!

The Diet was created by Dr. Arthur Agatston, a highly respected cardiologist, to work with your body safely and effectively. This diet works in phases, the first two for a specific timeframe and the third phase for life. With this new approach, you can stop counting calories, stop weighing food portions, and stop feeling as though you are deprived from eating good-tasting and satisfying food! Actually, you will be eating three, normal-size meals but wait, that not all! You will also get two snacks each day and with meal plans that are designed to be flexible, you can enjoy a variety, based on what sounds good to you on any particular day.

Best of all, you will see amazing results in a short amount of time. Your hips, thighs, and stomach will be thinner, the number on the scales will go down, and all those overwhelming food cravings will be gone! Just imagine losing weight while still enjoying many of your favourite foods. With the diet, you can dine on mouth-watering foods like Chicken en Papillote, Shrimp Louis, and even Chocolate Sponge Cake and still lose the weight!

South Beach Diet Phase

There are basically three phases in SB Diet. You eat normal portion sizes In Phase 1, but all carbohydrate are restricted. This is the strictest phase in the diet and will last for two weeks. It emphasizes lean meats, such as chicken, turkey, fish, and shellfish. Low-Glycemic-index vegetables are allowed as well as low-fat cheese, nuts, eggs. Dieters should expect to lose somewhere between 8 to 12 pounds. In Phase 2, some of the banned food are slowly introduced while weight loss continue to around 1-2 pounds per week. You should remain on it until you lost your desired amount of weight. Phase 3 is for maintenance and should be followed for life. Is all about maintaining your desired weight with a healthy balanced diet. Should your weight begin to climb, simply return to Phase 1.

The South Beach Diet emphasizes eating healthy carbohydrates, such as whole grains and certain fruits and vegetables, and healthy fats, such as olive and canola oil, and lean sources of protein. The diet is divided into three phases, with the initial 14-day phase being the most strict. The purpose of the first two weeks is to alter how your body responds to food. It is help you to overcome your food cravings and to eat fewer of the foods that cause your body to store excess fat. This weight loss diet requires no calorie count, no percentage count of fats, carbohydrates, and proteins, and no rules about portion sizes. Weight loss results are based on eating habits alone, not exercising, although regular exercise is of course recommended and can help speed up the weight loss process.

Phase 1 – Two Weeks
- Must eat three balanced meals per day, with mandatory snacks (such as nuts and low-fat cheese)
- Eat normal-size portions of lean meat, fish, eggs, reduced-fat cheese, nonfat yogurt, nuts, and vegetables.
- No bread, rice, potatoes, pasta, baked goods, fruit, candy, cakes, cookies, ice cream, sugar, beer, alcohol

Phase 2 – Length not specified (once you reach your goal weight)
Begin reintroducing healthy carbs, such as fruits and whole-grain breads and pastas (avoid white flour and white sugar). Choose a single carb and add it to one daily meal for a week. Continue this process until you are able to eat two to three servings of the rights carb a day.

Phase 3 – Life-long
Once you've reached your goal weight, you move to the maintenance phase, the stage that lasts for the rest of your life. Here you continue to make smart food choices, eating healthy carbs and fats.

A Sample Meal Plan in Phase 1 of the South Beach Diet
- Breakfast: two-egg omelette (may include some asparagus, broccoli, mushrooms, peppers, ham, low-fat cheese), two slices of Canadian bacon, cooked in a spray of olive or canola oil, coffee or tea if preferred, with low-fat milk and sugar substitute
- Snack: part-skim mozzarella stick
- Lunch: salad – lettuce, tomato mixed with grilled chicken or fish, dressed in a vinaigrette made with olive oil
- Snack: nuts (not salted or smoked) 15 almonds or cashews or 30 pistachios
- Dinner: Grilled salmon with lemon or roasted eggplant and a salad
- Dessert: sugar-free gelatin or tiramisu (made with low-fat ricotta, unsweetened cocoa powder, almonds, sugar substitute)

Sugar Busters

The Sugar Busters Diet is based on the premise that sugar can cause digestive problems, as well as being a major factor in weight gain. The authors say too much sugar causes the body to overproduce insulin, a hormone that regulates blood sugar levels and fat storage. Excess insulin production leads to increased amounts of body fat and weight, and stimulates the liver to make cholesterol.

The theory behind this diet is that by balancing the insulin-glucagon relationship in the body you'll lose body fat regardless of your calorie intake. Insulin is a hormone produced by the body to lower blood sugar when it gets too high, and glucagon is a hormone produced by the body to raise blood sugar when it goes too low.

How Sugar Busters Diet Works

The Sugar Busters Diet is easy to follow and, if you follow their 14-day diet exactly, you should lose weight. The plan is similar to those of many other low-carbohydrate plans: 40% carbohydrates, 30% protein, and 30% fat. The New Sugar Busters book mentions that you can increase carbohydrates to 50% as long as the choices are low-GI foods.

While on this diet, you are allowed to eat red meat, poultry, fish, olive oil, dairy foods, and nuts. There are certain fruits and vegetables you can eat as well. The authors of the diet claim that this diet discourages-and is in fact wary of-saturated fats, not only because they can cause weight gain, but because of the effect they can have upon vital organs, the heart in particular. They also advise that all meat should be lean and should have the fat trimmed off it. The authors recommend cooking with oils that are high in mono- and polyunsaturated fats and low in saturated fats, such as canola. High fibre foods are also encouraged in this diet, although some high fibre foods, such as bananas, are prohibited because they also contain high levels of sugar. As mentioned, you must also eliminate potatoes, corn, white rice, bread from refined flour, beets, carrots and, of course, refined sugar, corn syrup, molasses, honey, and sugared colas. Oats, small amounts of whole-grain bread, and whole-wheat pasta are also permitted. If you choose alcohol, you should drink red wine.

Advantages of Sugar Busters Diet
- The Sugar Busters Diet gives clear guidelines on which foods to avoid.
- The diet helps to eliminate consumption of refined sugar.

Disadvantages of Sugar Busters Diet
- The Sugar Busters Diet downplays the idea that calorie intake causes weight gain or weight loss.
- There is no scientific justification for the premise that healthy people who eat foods high in sugar will automatically gain weight.

Dieticians Comments About Sugar Busters Diet

Any diet that encourages high-fibre foods such as whole grains, fresh fruits, and vegetables in place of candy and refined flour products is applauded by nutritionists. However, when otherwise-healthy fruits and vegetables like pineapple, raisins, carrots, and bananas are restricted because they make blood sugar levels rise too quickly, you have to wonder about the logic of the diet. Also, the idea that sugar is toxic to the body is complete nonsense; although sugar has no nutritional value and counts as "empty calories," it is in no way toxic.

The most controversial claim of the Sugar Busters Diet is that insulin resistance can be reduced, by eliminating or severely restricting certain foods. Insulin resistance is a condition wherein our bodies have become insensitive to normal levels of circulating insulin in the bloodstream. Normally, a small amount of insulin will control blood sugar levels, but with insulin resistance, larger and larger amounts of insulin are pumped into the blood in an effort to lower blood sugar. Medical experts assert that the diet does not cause insulin resistance but that it is rather caused by obesity.

Sugar Busters, Sample menu 1

Breakfast:
Vegetable omelette and strawberries

Snack:
Cottage cheese, blueberries and walnuts

Lunch:
Balsamic glazed salmon
Broccoli sprinkled with olive oil, garlic and lemon juice
Brown rice

Dinner:
Dry rub BBQ chicken,
Couscous with almonds and spinach
Sliced fresh peach

Sugar Busters, Sample menu 2

Breakfast:
Scrambled eggs with spinach and cheese
Bowl of grapes

Snack:
Protein shake

Lunch:
Black bean soup
Fruit salad

Dinner:
Sauteed scallops with brown rice and raspberries

Volumetrics

The key to weight management with the Volumetrics Diet lies in the food choices that help you feel full with fewer calories. For more than 20 years, Barbara Rolls, Ph.D. has researched appetite and appetite control. The culmination of her research studies were published in a book, co-authored by Robert A. Barnett, The Volumetrics Weight-Control Plan. Rolls believes the absence of satiety, or the sensation of fullness, is one reason why most diets don't work very well or for very long. "The biggest mistake dieters make is that they eat less of everything, and then they feel hungry," says Rolls. Volumetrics is based on the concept of "energy density," which means how concentrated the calories are in a portion of food. High energy density foods provide a large number of calories in a small serving, while low energy density foods provide a small number of calories in a large serving.

Rolls contends that people need to eat more low-energy-dense (few calories per ounce) and a high-volume foods, such as fruits and vegetables, so they get that satisfying amount of food and enough calories. This view is echoed in the 2005 Dietary Guidelines for Americans. The secret ingredients that make foods less energy dense are water and fibre, which explains why most vegetables and fruits are among the lowest-energy foods. The higher the water content and/or the higher the fibre content, the lower the energy density of the food and the more volume the food has, which affects how full you feel. Keep fibre intake high, drink a lot of water, and eat a lot of foods high in water content and low in energy density, and you will lose weight. At the other end of the spectrum are the low-volume, energy-dense foods (which means they have a lot of calories per gram) such as chocolate chip cookies, ice cream, and nuts.

How Volumetrics Diet Works

There are no menus to follow and no mandates as to how or when certain foods should be eaten. Instead, Volumetrics contains extensive charts of the energy density (E.D.) and caloric content of any food group. One set of charts is broken down by the USDA Food Guide Pyramid food group and the other set provides listings for beverages, mixed dishes, fast foods, and desserts. The charts are arranged from lowest to highest energy density, making it easy to make good low-calorie, low-density choices. A low E.D. means you can eat more of the food; a high E.D. means you should restrict your intake. Although the charts are extensive, the E.D. of any food can be calculated by dividing the number of calories per serving by the weight in grams per serving.

Advantages of Volumetrics Diet
- Volumetrics helps you understand and overcome overeating without deprivation.
- There's a welcome emphasis on whole grains, fruits, and vegetables that is lacking in many diet plans.

Disadvantages of Volumetrics Diet
- The grocery bill for a Volumetrics Diet may be higher. On a per-calorie basis, fruits, vegetables, fish, lean protein, and low-fat diary products are more expensive sources of pure calories.
- People looking for a quick fix won't find it with this diet.

Dieticians Comments About Volumetrics Diet
Overall, the Volumetrics Diet receives good ratings from nutritionists because it encourages eating more fruits, vegetables, whole grains, legumes, and beans, and eating less high-fat, low-nutrient junk foods. If you have trouble controlling your weight and tend to overeat, the Volumetrics

weight control plan will help you eat less without deprivation. If you are true to the Volumetrics' formula for eating, you should feel satisfied and still lose weight.

Foods Allowed:
Focus on fibre-rich foods with a high moisture content. Fruits (mostly fresh), vegetables (mostly those with high water content; e.g. tomatoes, broccoli, greens) whole grain pasta, rice, breads and cereals; soups, salads; low-fat poultry, seafood, meats and dairy. Moderate amounts of sugar and alcohol are permitted, too.

Foods Restricted:
No foods are forbidden but limiting fatty foods like deep-fat fried items, sweets and fats added at the table are recommended. Limited amount of dry foods (crackers, popcorn, pretzels, etc.) due to their high caloric value and low satiety index.

Sample Menu:

Breakfast:
Oatmeal:
    1-1/3 cup oatmeal made with water
    1/2 medium apple
    1 teaspoon cinnamon
    2 teaspoons brown sugar
1 cup nonfat milk
1/2 grapefruit
Coffee

Lunch:
Grilled Chicken Salad:
    3ounces grilled chicken breast
    3 cups chopped Romaine lettuce
    4 slices red bell pepper
    2 tablespoons crumbled blue cheese
    1 tablespoon chopped walnuts
    2 tablespoons light dressing

1 whole wheat pita bread
1 cup sliced strawberries

Snack:
1 cup Cheerios
1/2 cup nonfat milk
2/3 cup fresh blueberries

Dinner:
Steak Fajita:
    3 ounces trimmed sirloin steak grilled
    1/2 cup grilled green pepper
    1/2 cup grilled onion

1 tablespoon reduced sodium soy sauce
2 tablespoons salsa
1/2 cup shredded Romaine lettuce
1/2 cup diced fresh tomato
2 tablespoons nonfat sour cream
1-10 inch flour tortilla
1/2 cup corn
1 cup diced cantaloupe

Waterfall Diet

There are many diet products and programs now on the market that claim to provide the secret to weight loss; one that usually requires very little effort on the part of the dieter. Weight loss is rarely that simple, and requires some patience and effort on the part of the dieter. Though, we believe that there are some useful weight loss tools available on the market.

The Waterfall Diet is a weight loss book written by Linda Lazarides, who has published a number of nutritional books. Though, this book in particular is said to show readers how to lose 14 pounds in just seven days. We will take a closer look at this book to determine the possible validity of this rather large claim.

According to the author, many doctors are unaware of the problems that water retention may cause. Lazarides believes that it may create tender breasts, painful and swollen joints, bloating and even the problem of excess fat. This book is meant to put dieters on a meal plan that will eliminate the problem of water retention and lead to a multitude of health benefits, and even weight loss.

However, we feel Lazarides does not adequately describe the science behind these statements, or why so many doctors are unaware of this rather common problem. The exact research she conducted to find these results are not shared online, and some dieters may not wish to read the entire book before seeing proof of her claims beforehand.

Diet Lifestyle

The diet plan that individuals of the Waterfall Diet will have to follow is not very clear. The author claims that there are seven different causes to water retention, and any person may have any one or two of these problems. In order to find out which problem a person has, they must complete a series of questionnaires that are provided in the book.

Some of the causes of water retention that the author cites include anaemia (anaemia), protein deficiency and an abnormally high need for one or more vitamins or minerals. She also says, "For women, hormonal changes prior to menstrual periods can also cause water retention. Producing extra hormones requires more nutrients, so mild premenstrual nutritional deficiencies are especially likely to occur at this time, and these can account for various unpleasant symptoms, including breast tenderness and tummy swelling."

Consumer Feedback

We are unable to find much feedback about this diet online. We are unsure if this means that the results of the program are so uninspiring that people do not bother to share them online, or if few people are interested enough to even try the diet. However, we know that testimonials are often valuable in gauging the potential success rate of a supplement or a program. Some people may prefer to use products or plans that display many varied testimonials on the product website.

Positives
 May solve the problem of water retention for some
 Book may be found at reduced prices

Negatives
 May not offer a proven way to approach weight loss

Offers no guidance on how to suppress the appetite
May not burn off significant fat
May advertise unrealistic results

Dieters who have gained success on another of Lazarides' nutrition books may be interested in trying the Waterfall Diet. Though, we wonder how solving the problem of water retention may lead to 14 pounds of weight loss in just seven days. If this diet works, we believe it may just address excess water weight and not actual fat.

Many dieters are most interested in losing fat so that they may decrease their risk of developing dangerous health conditions that are linked with obesity. Those people who feel that this diet may not provide significant enough results may prefer to look into an herbal capsule-based formula that contains Hoodia, which is an herb proven to reduce hunger and aid with portion control.

The Diet is divided into 3 parts:

Phase 1
Fluid retention sufferers are recommended to follow this phase for 2 months. It is designed to help clear your system of residues which may be encouraging fluid retention, and to provide the necessary raw materials for building up the strength of your capillaries and balancing your electrolytes, hormones and prostaglandins. This phase is strict because this gets you the clearest and most rapid results.

- Avoid even small amounts of the Banned Foods list.
- Consume the Allowed Foods as frequently as possible
- Balance foods to ensure the greatest possible variety.

Phase 2
This phase takes 4 weeks. It is similar to Phase I, but involves testing yourself for food allergies / intolerances which may have been contributing to your fluid retention.

Test yourself for the following food:

- **Wheat**: bread, flour, biscuits, sauces, puddings
- **Dairy**: milk, cream, cheese, yoghurt, butter
- **Yeast**: alcoholic drinks, stock cubes, gravy mix, bread, pizza
- **Egg**: egg dishes, egg pasta, ice cream, desserts, batter, pancakes

If you lost a lot of fluid within a few days during Phase I, it is 90% likely that you have an allergy or intolerance to one of these 4 foods. The only way to find out for sure is to reintroduce these foods into your diet one by one in a carefully controlled way. That is what this phase is all about.

Phase 3
This phase is more relaxed, and allows you a wide variety of foods. It is less a diet and more a long term eating strategy, encouraging you to be conscious of foods that promote or fight your specific type of fluid retention and to eat accordingly.

The Banned Foods are no longer unconditionally forbidden. You may resume them, subject to 2 conditions:

- That you continue to avoid the specific foods which aggravate your particular type of fluid retention.
- 90% of your diet should continue to consist of whole grains and unrefined foods, fruit and vegetables and their juices, nuts and seeds, tofu and other soya products, and 'oily' fish.

FOOD LISTS

Allowed foods

Apples, avocados, bananas, beans, beetroot, bilberries, blueberries, blackberries, black grapes, black cherries, broccoli, brussels sprouts, cabbage, carrots, cauliflower, celery, dried fruit, eggs, salmon, herring, mackerel, pilchards, white fish, gelatine, lentils, liver, sheep milk, goat's milk, nuts, seeds, olive oil, onions, orange, lemon, fruit, parsley, peanuts, peppers, horseradish, porridge oats, potatoes, brown rice, soya flour, soya milk, tofu, tomatoes, vegetables, soy yoghurt, free range chicken

Banned foods

Coffee, sugar, honey, syrup, foods containing added sugar, salt, salted / smoked food, salami, ham, bacon, smoked fish, salty cheeses, stock cubes, yeast extract, soy sauce, baking powder, soft drinks, fat, burgers, sausages, pork pies, chocolate, crisps, fried food, butter, margarine, cream, cheese, mayonnaise, pastry, white flour, alcohol, artificial food additives, wheat, bread, pasta, dairy, eggs, yeast, red meat, batter, cheese, ice cream, yoghurt

Avoid that lot and you are almost certain to be reducing your calorie intake significantly even if you eat your fill of the non-banned foods, which include soya milk and yoghurt, fruit, vegetables, seeds, nuts, oats, brown rice, pulses, lean organic poultry and fish. To drink you can have water, home made juices, herb teas, and other low-caffeine drinks.

Approximate calorie content - 1,000 calories a day.

PROS
- There is no portion control, so you can eat all you want of the allowed foods, which should keep you feeling full as there is plenty of fibre and foods low on the Glycaemic Index.
- Can lose up to 14 pounds in a week.
- If you shop wisely, choosing fruit and vegetables in season and the cheaper items like pulses and tofu, it needn't be too expensive. Also you will not be buying all those added-value foods like cakes, or alcohol.
- Avoiding all foods which may encourage fluid retention - particularly refined carbohydrates and salt - will cause the body to lose several pounds of fluid, though the amount will vary from person to person. Some body fat will also be lost.

CONS
- Looking for healthy alternatives that are not commonly available, e.g. potassium salt, can be time consuming and more expensive than the average product in its range.
- The diet has the potential to be quite a healthy one though items such as wholemeal bread are banned at first as are lean red meat, whole wheat pasta, eggs and cheese - all staples in most people's diets, and all good foods as part of a balanced diet. This may cause nutritional imbalances over time unless you're very careful.
- There are plenty of fruit and vegetables and the diet is very low in saturated fat but the

tone of the diet tends to encourage faddy eating.

- For the Western palate, this will be a shock. But if it is persisted with, the palate should change and the fresh flavours of this basically natural diet should begin to win.
- For most people who have been eating a typical Western diet, this diet would be particularly hard to adapt to; major changes need to be made.
- The diet is likely to continue to produce weight loss and there is a long term strategy explained, but for many people we fear it will be hard to stick to this diet for life.

Weight Watchers

Probably the most recognized of the organized weight loss programs, Weight Watchers, founded by Dr. Jean Nidetch, has been around since a humble beginning in Queens, New York, in 1963. Though Weight Watchers has changed a lot over the years, it has remained steadfast in its goal of offering weight loss guidance in a group support environment while emphasizing a balanced diet and encouraging exercise. At local group meetings, Weight Watchers' members get motivation, mutual support and encouragement in handling the challenges encountered in the process of changing behaviour.

Weight Watchers has produced its own line of cuisine, which may be purchased independently at most major grocery chains. There is a one-time registration fee and a weekly fee.

How Weight Watchers Diet Works

The Weight Watchers program is based on calorie reduction using the Weight Watchers Points system. Foods are assigned a certain number of points according to their calorie count, the number of fat grams they contain, and their fibre content. The higher the fat grams the more points assigned to that food. The higher the fibre grams the fewer the points assigned to that food. Dieters are allotted a certain number of points, referred to as the Daily Point Range, that is determined by their body weight and the number of pounds they want to lose. Dieters must record all foods eaten and their point value every day to make sure they're staying within their assigned points. Stay within the Daily Points Range and you'll lose weight. The number of points each dieter is allotted daily ranges from 18 to 35 points, which is based on their body weight, and how much weight they are trying to lose. For example, a 5'6" woman who weights 180 pounds would be allotted between 22 and 27 points each day.

Weight Watchers is extremely flexible about the foods you can eat; in fact, you can literally eat anything and lose weight, so long as you keep track of your points and don't exceed your Daily Point Range. For example, one cup of grapes counts as one point, one scoop of ice cream as four points, and one slice of pizza as nine points. The more points you use on a single item, the fewer foods you'll be able to eat during the day. Although the choices are left to the dieter, Weight Watchers leaders and materials offer considerable guidance for choosing a healthy and nutritious diet.

Advantages of Weight Watchers Diet
- Dieters participating in the Weight Watchers program generally lose as much weight as those who used their own do it-yourself approach.
- The group support the Weight Watchers program provides is one of its strongest features.

Disadvantages of Weight Watchers Diet
- The Weight Watchers Points system can be abused. Someone could potentially spend a whole day's points on ice cream or junk food.
- Calorie counting does raise our awareness of the relative caloric value of foods. However, calorie content is only one standard of measurement. A candy bar may contain the same calories/points as a large sandwich, but it's not as healthy or nutritious.

Dieticians Comments About Weight Watchers Diet

Overall, the Weight Watchers Diet generally receives good ratings from nutritionists because its emphasis is on moderate fat and balanced nutrients. Typically, people who follow the Weight Watchers Points program over a period of time will lose weight. While, on average, participants lost only small amounts of weight while enrolled in the structured Weight Watchers Points program, some participants can lose considerably more weight, with the maximum amount of weight loss reaching about 50 pounds. Many believe the structured program has its advantages over trying to lose the weight on your own.

Sample Weight Watchers Menu

A day on Weight Watchers' Core Plan might look like this:

Breakfast:
- Vegetables scrambled with egg whites, or cup of bran flakes with skim milk
- Cup of berries
- Fat-free yogurt
- Tea

Lunch:
- Cup of vegetable soup
- Black-bean burger or turkey on whole-grain bread with lettuce and tomato
- Slice of melon
- Water

Dinner:
- Big green salad
- Four slices of pork tenderloin
- Steamed zucchini and summer squash
- Half a cup of brown rice
- Cup of fruit smoothie

Snacks:
- Most vegetables and fruits
- Lean protein such as a slice of chicken or turkey
- Cup or two of air-popped or light popcorn

Zone Diet

It comes from the Greek root meaning "way of life". This is what the Zone Diet is. It's a way of life to help control gene expression to give you the longer and better life we all aspire to.

The Zone Diet gives you the power to turn some genes on and turn other genes off. As a result, you feel your energy soar, watch your waistline shrink, and say goodbye to hunger. In the Zone you are now taking wellness into your own hands.

Any diet that uses the word high or low to describe it is hormonally unsustainable. The only diet that can maintain hormonal balance for a lifetime must use the word moderate to describe it. That's what the Zone Diet is.

It's moderate in:

> Low-fat protein
> Low glycemic-load carbs(mostly fruits and vegetables)
> Heart-healthy monounsaturated fats

The Zone Diet is about balancing your hormones within a specific range to control hunger on fewer calories while still getting the proper nutrients your body needs for long-term health. The Zone Diet can best be described as a moderate-carbohydrate, moderate-protein, moderate fat diet that has approximately one gram of fat for every two grams of protein and three grams of carbohydrates. These ratios represent the newest dietary recommendations from the Joslin Diabetes Research Centre at Harvard Medical School for the treatment of obesity and type 2 diabetes.

With the right balance of protein, carbohydrates and fats, you can control three major hormones generated by the diet – insulin, glucagon and eicosanoids.

Insulin – A storage hormone. Excess insulin makes you fat and keeps you fat.

Glucagon – A mobilization hormone that tells the body to release stored carbohydrates at a steady rate, leading to stabilized blood sugar levels. This is key for optimal mental and physical performance.

Eicosanoids – They are master hormones that indirectly orchestrate a vast array of other hormonal systems in your body.

'Enter the Zone' and you'll lose weight permanently, achieve peak physical performance, enhance mental productivity and delay the signs of ageing. At least that's what Barry Sears, creator of The Zone Diet, tells us!

In the mid 1990's, the Zone was all the rage with many celebs, all claiming to be fans of the plan. Before long, millions of people were following the Zone and the diet had become a household name. Now, even though newer diet plans such as the Atkins and South Beach Diets gain more column inches and their books currently head the New York Times Bestseller list, the Zone Diet continues to remain a popular choice for some.

What's the theory?

The Zone Diet works on the theory that excess insulin, a hormone that helps control our blood sugar levels, makes us fat and keeps us fat. By closely regulating our blood sugar levels and therefore keeping our levels of insulin in a tight 'zone', the body burns fat more efficiently so that we lose weight.

To control blood sugar levels and consequently insulin levels, you need to get the perfect balance of carbohydrates, proteins and fats in every meal. Achieving this perfect balance effectively means following a low-carbohydrate, high-protein diet that includes moderate amounts of fat. And if that sounds familiar, you'd be right! In fact, the Zone Diet is not too dissimilar to many of the other low-carb, high-protein diets that are currently in vogue, either in terms of the theory or the foods you can and can't eat.

What does the Zone Diet involve?

If the theory sounds simple, the reality is far more complicated. First off, you'll need plenty of patience, a head for science and the desire to learn more about 'zoning', either by looking at the Zone website or indulging in some bedtime reading, courtesy of creator Barry Sears.

The idea is that to reach 'The Zone', every meal and snack should provide 40 percent of calories from carbohydrate, 30 per cent from protein and 30 per cent from fat. This is what some Zone fans call the 40:30:30 ratio.

To help with this, 'Zone Food Blocks' have been developed, where each 'block' contains a standardised amount of carbohydrate, protein or fat. To lose weight, a certain number of blocks are allocated for each meal and snack.

The number of Zone Food Blocks you should have each day is calculated according to your weight, height and waist and hip circumferences. Generally, the bigger you are, the more blocks you are allowed. For example, a woman who weighs 10st, is 5ft 2in, has a 28in waist and 37in hips should have 12 blocks a day (four for breakfast, three each for lunch and dinner, one for an afternoon snack and one for an evening snack). Meanwhile, a larger woman who weighs 12st, is 5ft 10in, has a 30in waist and 40in hips needs 14 blocks (four for each main meal and one each as an afternoon snack and an evening snack).

With help from Weight Loss Resources or the Zone's website, Zone Perfect, calculating the daily number of blocks you should have – and how they should be divided throughout the day – is the easy bit. Creating meals and snacks that have the correct number of Zone Foods Blocks is the hard bit! No surprises then that you really need a Zone Diet book to help you put meals together. And if that's still too much like hard work, there are many pre-packaged Zone Diet meals and snacks for delivery that you can order over the Internet – at a fairly hefty price!

This sounds like hard work! Is there an easier way to follow it?

Although the creator of the diet is quite adamant that for best effects you should really stick to counting Food Blocks, it's still possible to follow the basic principles of the diet without going through this complicated process.

In simple terms, the Zone diet involves cutting out most carbohydrates such as breakfast cereals, rice, potatoes, pasta, noodles, bread, bagels, croissants, muffins, crisps, pastries, pies, chocolate, sweets, sugar and preserves, as these have the greatest effect on blood sugar levels and therefore insulin levels. Most fruit and vegetables, however, are allowed. Low-fat protein-rich foods such as skinless chicken, turkey and fish should be eaten with every meal. Meanwhile, eating fewer foods that contain saturates and choosing foods that are rich in monounsaturates, such as olive oil, avocado and nuts, is recommended.

To make the Zone Diet even easier to follow, the creator recommends dividing your plate into three equal sized sections and then filling one section with low-fat protein such as chicken – making sure it's no larger or thicker than the palm of your hand – and the remaining two sections with vegetables and fruit. Adding a little olive oil, avocado or a few nuts will help to boost intakes of monounsaturates!

So how much weight can I expect to lose?

Advocates of the Zone Diet claim you can lose at least 5lb in the first two weeks, followed by 1-1.5lb every week after this.

What do the experts say?

Achieving a 40:30:30 ratio is certainly a departure from current healthy eating guidelines, which recommend 50 percent of our calories should come from carbohydrate, 15 percent from protein and 35 percent from fat. While most nutrition experts agree with the advice to eat less fat, especially saturates, and to fill up on fruit and veg, most remain sceptical about the theory that weight loss is due to regulating insulin levels. They still believe that eating fewer carbohydrate-rich foods results in a calorie deficit – in other words, any weight loss that occurs is due to taking in fewer calories than the body uses up. In fact, if followed properly, the diet provides around 1,000 to 1,300 calories a day, thanks mainly to cutting out most high-calorie sugary and starchy foods – and replacing them with low-calorie vegetables and fruit. And if you're still not convinced, maybe this example will help: swap a large Danish pastry, containing around 650 calories, for a 50-calorie apple and you'll save a staggering 600 calories. Do this every day for a week and you'd expect to lose more than 1lb in a week!

Are there any pros?
The Zone Diet generally has fewer dietary restrictions than many other low-carb plans and recommends eating more fruit and vegetables. It also encourages you to cut out a lot of the 'junk' or low-nutrient carbs in your diet such as crisps, cakes, biscuits and chocolate. Eating fewer fatty foods – and swapping foods that are high in saturates for those containing monounsaturates – is sensible, heart-healthy advice, too.

And the cons?
Unfortunately, the Zone Diet is very complicated and time-consuming if you're going to follow it properly. You'll need to invest in a Zone diet book and a decent set of measuring scales and spoons if you don't already have them. It also recommends eliminating some very nutritious foods, which are not only a good source of carbohydrate but are also packed with fibre and important vitamins and minerals. For example, wholegrain cereals are packed with fibre, B vitamins and iron, while cheese is an excellent source of calcium and zinc. It can also be really expensive if you decide to purchase pre-packaged Zone products

Getting Ready To Make Zone Meals
Ironically, the Zone is based on two terms your grandmother told you: balance and moderation. You balance your plate at every meal, and never eat too many calories at a meal. The only tools you need are the palm of your hand and your eye.

Start With Protein
Every Zone meal starts with making sure that you have an adequate serving of low-fat protein. There are several reasons for this. The first is that your body needs a constant supply of dietary protein to replace the protein that is constantly lost from your body on a daily basis. Without adequate incoming protein, your muscles weaken and your immune system becomes far less effective. Second, protein stimulates the release of glucagons. Glucagon is a mobilization hormone that tells the body to release stored carbohydrates from the liver to maintain adequate blood sugar levels for the brain. Without adequate protein in a meal, hunger (due to the inability to maintain blood sugar levels) will result in two to three hours after a meal. Finally, glucagon acts as a brake on excess insulin secretion. If glucagon levels increase, then insulin levels decrease. By stimulating the release of enough glucagon with adequate levels of protein, you now have an ideal control mechanism to prevent too much insulin from being released.

Finally, you always want to use low-fat protein. Why? Because you will always be adding a dash of monounsaturated fat to a Zone meal, and using low-fat protein means you can control the composition of your fat instead of overconsuming saturated fat.

A very common misconception about the Zone is that you have to eat animal protein. That's simply not true. You do have to consume adequate protein, but for a vegetarian that is very easy to achieve eating egg whites, low-fat dairy products, tofu, or soy meat substitutes. Using soy products as your primary protein source may actually be the healthiest version of the Zone for a longer life. The first step of Zone meal preparation is to never consume any more low-fat protein at a meal than you can fit on the palm of your hand. And before you get too excited, that amount also means the thickness of your hand. For most American females, this is 3 ounces of low-fat protein, and for most American males this is about 4 ounces of low-fat protein. Unless you are very active, your body can't utilize any more protein than that at a single sitting: any excess protein will be converted to fat. You always want to use low-fat protein for Zone meals to keep the amount of saturated fat to a minimum (since it can indirectly increase insulin levels). What are some good sources of low-fat protein? Many of your best choices follow.

Best Protein Choices
Skinless chicken
Turkey
Fish
Very lean cuts of meat
Egg whites
Low-fat dairy products
Tofu
Soy meat substitutes

Balance With Carbohydrates
Now that you have your protein portion for your Zone meal, you must balance the protein with carbohydrates. Unfortunately, most Americans have no idea what carbohydrates actually are. Many people think of them as only pasta and sweets, whereas in reality they also include fruits and vegetables. The fact that a fruit or vegetable is also a carbohydrate is a major revelation to most Americans. However, not all carbohydrates are equal in their ability to stimulate insulin. Some are "favourable" carbohydrates that have a low capacity to stimulate insulin, and others are "unfavourable" carbohydrates that have a high capacity to stimulate insulin. Since the name of the game is insulin control, you want to make sure that most of your carbohydrate choices come from favourable carbohydrates (primarily fruits and vegetables), and treat unfavourable carbohydrates (such as grains and starches) like condiments.

This definition of favourable and unfavourable is based on the concept of the glycemic load. That is calculated from the combination of both the density of the carbohydrate in a given volume, and the rate at which it will enter the bloodstream. More details about glycemic load are found Dr. Sears' book The Zone, but for now all you need to know is that the higher the glycemic load of a given volume of carbohydrate, the greater its ability to stimulate insulin.

Vegetables (except for corn and carrots) always have a low glycemic load, whereas fruits (except for bananas and raisins) will usually have an intermediate glycemic load. Starches and grains (except for oatmeal and barley, which are very rich in soluble fibre) have very high glycemic loads. Therefore, as you balance the protein on your plate, do so with a lot of vegetables, some fruits, and just a small amount of grains and starches. Here are some of the favourable and unfavourable carbohydrates.

Favourable Carbohydrates
Most vegetables (except corn and carrots)
Most fruits (except bananas & raisins)

Selected grains (oatmeal and barley)

Unfavourable Carbohydrates
Grains and starches (pasta, bread, bagels, cereals, potatoes, etc.)
Selected fruits (bananas, raisins, etc.)
Selected vegetables (corn and carrots)
As you can readily see, a good portion of your current diet is probably heavy on large amounts of unfavourable carbohydrates without adequate levels of low-fat protein. That's a surefire prescription for elevated insulin, which means you are getting fatter and less healthy with each meal.

Add Fat
Once you have balanced your plate with low-fat protein and favourable carbohydrates, there is one more thing to add before it's truly a Zone meal – fat. Remember, it takes fat to burn fat. But like carbohydrates, all fats are not equal.
There are two types of fats that fall into the category of "good fats". These are monounsaturated fats and long-chain omega-3 fats. You get monounsaturated fats from olive oil, selected nuts, and avocados. Long-chain omega-3 fats come from fish and fish oils (like the cod liver oil your grandmother told you to take). These are exceptionally powerful allies in your quest for a longer life.
However, there are some fats you want to restrict in your diet. These are saturated fats, trans fats, and arachidonic acid. I consider these to be really "bad" fats. You find saturated fats in fatty cuts of red meat and high-fat dairy products. Another type of fat to avoid is trans fats. These artificial fats were created by the food industry. Any time you see the words "partially hydrogenated vegetable oil," you know that food contains trans fats. These alien fats make processed food more stable. Furthermore, Harvard Medical School has shown that the more trans fats you eat, the more at risk you are for heart disease. Finally there is arachidonic acid, which is found primarily in fatty red meats, egg yolks, and organ meats.
This particular polyunsaturated fat may be the most dangerous fat known when consumed in excess. In fact, you can inject virtually every type of fat (even saturated fat and cholesterol) into rabbits, and nothing happens. However, if you inject arachidonic acid into the same rabbits, they are dead within three minutes. The human body needs some arachidonic acid, but too much can be toxic. Ironically, the higher your insulin levels, the more your body is stimulated to make increased levels of arachidonic acid.

Good Fats
Olive oil
Almonds
Avocados
Fish oils

Bad Fats
Fatty red meat
Egg yolks
Organ meats
Processed foods (rich in trans fats)

Lets Get Started

Now that you have an idea of what types of protein, carbohydrate, and fat you will be using to make Zone meals, here is how easy it really is.

First, take your plate and divide it into three sections. On one-third of the plate put some low-fat protein that is no bigger or thicker than the palm of your hand. Then fill the other two-thirds of the plate until it is overflowing with fruits and vegetables. Then a dash (that's a small amount) of monounsaturated fat, like olive oil, slivered almonds, or even guacamole. There you have it: a Zone meal.

You can see that putting together a Zone meal isn't rocket science. But the key is consistency, since the hormonal benefits of each meal will only last four to six hours. You have to eat, so you might as well get the best hormonal bang for the buck out of each meal.

This means always balancing protein and carbohydrate at every meal and snack. For example, you can't have all of your protein in one meal and all of your carbohydrate in the next meal, because your insulin levels will swing all over the place. Consider your food like a medication. You have to take the right dose at the right time. Would you take a week's worth of drugs on Saturday afternoon? Of course not. And if you are taking your drug every day, would you take 5 mg in the morning, 500mg at noon, and 28mg in the evening? Of course not. You would try the best you could to take the same amount of the drug each time. Why? You want to keep the drug within a Zone; not too high (where it's toxic), nor too low (where it doesn't work). Treat food the same way. Your goal is to maintain insulin in a similar Zone by balancing protein and carbohydrate and using only your eye and the palm of your hand to do it.

Appendix 2

50 Muscle Building Tips

Contents

26. Low Fat

27. Eat Well And Often

28. Balanced Diet

29. Water

30. Be Consistent

31. Take A Break

32. Vitamins And Minerals

33. Creatine

34. Glutamine

35. MSM

36. Supplements

37. Choose Your Time

38. Stick To The Program

39. Create A Balanced Life

40. Rest

41. Sleep

42. Patience

43. Stress

44. Alcohol

45. Illness

46. Trial And Error

47. Confidence

48. Positive Mental Attitude

49. Take A Break

50. Long Term Goals

Introduction

50 Muscle Building Tips will help you improve your results from any training program.

Whether you are just running, working out at home, going to the gym or training for competitions you will find some useful tips and advice in the following pages.

This report can be read as a book from start to finish or you could use it as a reference work which you dip in and out of for particular sections.

The basic information which you will find in here can be supplemented by further reading with specialised books on the subjects you are most interested in.

1. Warming Up

After 'warming up' your body is ready to exercise. It is an essential aspect of training as it prepares your body for the more strenuous exercises to follow.

Your heart rate, body temperature and metabolic rate will all increase when you warm up. This means that your body is not working 'from cold'. It is exactly the same concept with motor cars. When you start an engine, the engine oil is heated up and pumped around the engine, and the engine works better after the oil has been heated up.

When your body has been warmed up, your blood will flow faster which in turn makes sure that a constant supply of oxygen is being taken to all of your muscles which is vital when such demands are being placed on them during exercising.

Another very important reason to warm up is that it reduces the chances of injury. When your body and muscles are warmed up, they operate much better and are less likely to be strained.

Start with a general body warm up. This is done before any exercise session and can consist of 10 minutes of running on the spot, stationary bike, rowing or even simply going up and down stairs to get your heart rate going and warming up the muscles.

Before each specific exercise, it is also advisable to complete a warm up which will target that muscle or muscle group which you are about to exercise. This will help to improve the flexibility of the targeted areas and allow them to work at a greater level of intensity.

An additional form of warm up is the exercise specific warm up. This takes the form of the actual exercise which you are about to perform but without using any weights or putting any strain onto the muscle. Do the exercise in a gentle form simply to get the muscles used to the form of the exercise.

After these warm ups, you will then be ready to achieve the greatest level of return from each exercise.

2. Stretching Your Muscles

Stretching your muscles helps to increase the flexibility of your muscles.

Along with flexibility, a slow stretch or static stretch will help to reduce immediate muscle soreness and increase the muscle's range of movement.

Stretching should release tension from the muscle which is why you must not stretch a muscle too far otherwise you risk straining the muscle. Stretch a little to start with and as your muscles become used to this, they will begin to be more flexible and you will be able to stretch further.

Not a great deal of stretching is required. Do it for ten to fifteen seconds for each muscle before you exercise that particular muscle.

Stretching does not need to add to the length of your workout either. You can stretch for the next exercise while you are in your rest period from your previous exercise. This is an excellent way to move from one exercise to the next.

3. Motivation By Visualisation

When you are exercising, you need to keep up your level of motivation. Without this continuous motivation, you will simply stop training and lose all the benefits which you have built up.

One way to help with motivation is by visualisation.

Imagine yourself going through your program.
Imagine yourself working really hard at al the exercises.
Imagine your muscles responding positively to the exercises.
Imagine your muscles growing bigger and bigger.
Imagine how you will feel, looking at your toned body in a mirror.

Top athletes use these techniques to increase their performance. When a 100 meter sprinter is preparing for a race, they will have 'run' the race many times in their head before getting anywhere near the track. They will have imagined they are running at peak performance. They will have imagined winning the race.

There are lots of images you can create in your mind which can positively motivate you to continue with your training. Use your mind and imagination as a training tool. It is not just about the weights.

4. Target Specific Muscles

To make the most gains in strength, fitness and muscle mass you must target muscles and muscle groups rather than trying to work too many muscles at once.

When you start training, it is easy to complete all exercises within one session. When you become more advanced, you will need to target muscles more specifically to still make gains.

When you first start using targeting routines it will probably be one day for targeting your upper body muscles and on the following day you would be targeting your lower body muscles.

Targeting workouts in this way means that you can really push your upper body muscles on day one and then rest those same muscles on day two while you target your lower body muscles.

5. The Most Important Exercise

Many experts will tell you that the most important exercise in building a muscular body is the squat.

This exercise is a great exercise for your legs but it also conditions your whole body at the same time. Your leg muscles are the largest muscles in your body so targeting these muscles can really improve your overall condition.

Another reason for concentrating on squats is that they have been scientifically proven to be the exercise which releases more testosterone into your body. Testosterone helps to promote muscle growth, strength and puts extra power into your workout.

Make sure you spend time getting the form and technique of your squats just right to make sure you are getting the most out of this most important exercise.

6. Fully Work Each Muscle

You will make more gains in muscle size and strength if you take each muscle through its full range of motion. Stopping just slightly short of a full range of movement can reduce the effectiveness of an exercise quite dramatically and so this is vitally important to make maximum gains from your effort.

Make sure each exercise takes the muscle from its fully stretched position to its fully contracted position. As an example, when completing a bicep curl you should make sure the arm is fully stretched and as you lift the weight, you should make sure that you use your bicep to lift the weight through the full motion until you really feel the intensity within your bicep.

When you are working each muscle to both extremes, you should also concentrate on the form of the exercise to make absolutely sure that you can not get even a little more range of motion out of the exercise.

If you find it hard to complete an exercise with its full range of movement in one swift motion you can complete it in two sections. Using the bicep curl as an example again you should lift to just over half of the range of motion, slightly lower the arm, and then continue with the bicep curl to finish off the full range of movement for the muscle.

7. Hold At Maximum Intensity

To achieve greatest gains from your body building efforts you should know where you are able to reap the most rewards for your efforts.

When you are going through an exercise you will know where you feel the most intensity. This is where the muscle is working hardest. When the muscle is working at its maximum intensity you should hold the position for a second or two just to make sure the muscle is really working hard.

Moving to the position of maximum intensity, holding the position for a second or two and then moving out of the position of maximum intensity should all be done in a smooth flow. There should be no sudden jerks of the muscle as this can release the tension in the muscle with a resulting loss of opportunity for greater results.

Make sure that you do not use other muscles in your body to force the position of the muscle you are targeting. The form of your exercise should still remain perfect while you are holding for maximum intensity. Any loss of form will also result in the loss of achievable maximum results.

8. Reduce Rest Between Sets

Normally you would take a while between sets to fully recover. By reducing the amount of time you take to recover between sets you will increase the intensity of successive sets.

Reducing your resting period between completed sets will help to increase the long term growth of your muscles as they will respond with greater growth over time.

Some rest is definitely required between sets to make sure that your muscles short-term recovery is complete but resting for too long a period can hold back the progress in muscle growth which you can achieve.

There is a fine line which you must discover for your own particular body when it comes to rest. Too much rest between sets can hold you back but equally too little rest can mean that your muscles are not being given sufficient recovery time before they are being worked again. This is something you will have to test with trial and error until you achieve your optimum rest period.

Along with increasing the intensity of each exercise you will also reduce the amount of time spent exercising if you reduce your rest period lengths.

9. Increase Intensity

Muscles make gains in size and strength when they are pushed to their maximum force-generating capacity. Continually pushing your muscles to their maximum is when you will make most progress. The mechanism of pushing your muscles to this level is technically known as the overload principal.

You will exercise with an intensity where the weight being lifted can be completed about 8 or 10 times in a set. When you are using the same weight but start to reach 12 or 15 reps, this means that your muscle strength has increased and you should now increase the intensity of the exercise by loading the weight so that the number of reps you can complete is reduced again to 8 or 10 reps. By continually increasing the weight or intensity of each exercise in this way, you will continually increase the strength and sizes of your muscles.

By keeping the maximum reps you can complete at each intensity level to 8 or 10, you will be keeping your muscles working at the optimum level for muscle growth. You would gain size if you continued to work at level which allowed you to complete 15 reps but the increase in muscle mass would not be any where near as big an increase as continually reducing the reps you could manage by continually increasing the weights or intensity of the exercises.

10. Work With Your Muscles

You must work with your muscles rather than against them to achieve the best results. Nature has designed your body with its bones, muscles and tendons to work in a particular way to achieve the most efficient use of energy and power. Do not fight natures design but rather work with it.

Make sure that you train your muscles in the planes, directions and angles which they were designed to work in. Exercising muscles at odd angles which they were not designed for will not stimulate more growth or change the shape of your muscles.

Trying to train in unusual positions and awkward angles will also dramatically increase the risk of injury to yourself which would mean you would be out of action and not able to train at all.

Your muscles are connected to your bones with tendons and the positions of these connections can not be changed which means that the angles and positions that muscles should be worked can also not be changed.

If you try and push your body while it is in an unusual position you may feel some pain or an unusual sensation. These warning signs are the defence mechanism of your body telling you that you should not be training in this position or you should not be using a particular muscle in that angle. You must learn to listen to the warning signs of your body or you risk serious injury.

11. Using Isometrics

Isometric exercises can help to boost the gains in muscle mass and strength by providing another stimulus for muscle growth.

After completing a set of your standard exercises you should maintain isometric tension for about fifteen to twenty seconds remembering not to hold your breath while you hold the isometric position.

An isometric exercise is one where the muscle is contracted against an immovable object. An example of this would be when you force your palms together with one hand pushing down while the other hand pushes up against each other.

Try this exercise in different variations to get an idea of how to perform isometric exercises. With one arm held as though you are half way through a bicep curl, your palm facing up. Now place your other palm face down so that both palms are facing each other. Push both palms together and you will be able to feel the tension in your bicep. To work the other bicep, turn your palms over and try again.

Another isometric exercise would be to hold your hands out in front of you and rather than face up and face down, have them face each other as though you were clapping. Force them together and you will be able to feel your pectoral muscles being worked.

12. Using A Spotter

A spotter or a training partner can help increase the intensity of your workouts for a number of reasons.

You are able to help each other out by encouraging you to make those last few reps which you may have otherwise thought you just could not complete but with someone there shouting you on, you just manage to push yourself that little bit harder.

Choosing the correct spotter or partner can be a very important decision. You need someone who is reliable and will not leave you waiting there all the time for them to turn up or at worst not even turn up at all. This would quickly waste your time and completely destroy any motivation you had to push yourself. Even though you need someone who is reliable, there will be times when everyone has unavoidable reasons why they can not make appointments and you both will have to realise that there will be times when both your diaries do not match up or you have to let one another down on the odd occasion.

Equally, you would have to be reliable for the other person as it is a two way relationship. They would push you through your exercises and you would push them through theirs.

Pushing each other that bit further would mean that better gains would be achieved by both of you which should then lead to better motivation to keep up with the training program.

13. Push Yourself Hard

You will not make gains in either muscle mass or muscle strength if you just coast along in a training program. You have to be prepared to push yourself hard if you want to make any appreciable gains.

There will be times that you do not feel like training but if a session has been arranged and it is part of the program then you really do have to make the effort to complete it.

Much of the battle with training is in the mind. You have to have the right mindset to be able to complete training programs to the required level. Focus hard on how you can motivate yourself to complete all the exercises required. There are sections in this book which will help with that.

People who do a few exercises on a weights machine with low weights on them while chatting to their mate are not the people who are going to make any real gains. The people who are going to be really successful at building muscles are the ones who are focused, pushing high levels of weights while concentrating on what they are doing rather than being distracted by what is going on around them in the gym.

Set yourself some tough goals and make sure you stick to them. If you decide you are not going to bother pushing yourself then there is nobody who can make you. It is your decision and something you should think hard about.

14. Setting Goals

Goals are a good way of giving yourself specific targets which you can aim for and judge yourself against whether you achieve the results or whether you start to miss targets on a regular basis.

Beating targets can increase your confidence but only if the targets are meaningful. If the targets are too easy to beat then they are not something which you have to push yourself hard for. Equally, they should not be too hard to reach that you will continually be disheartened when you keep missing your own targets. Sometimes you will beat them which will boost your confidence but other times you will miss the targets which should be a wake up call that you will just have to push yourself harder the next time.

Set yourself different levels of targets. Short, medium and long term targets give you different aspects of goal setting to aim for.

Short term targets should be easily achievable so that you feel victory on a regular basis which will give you confidence to carry on.

Medium and long term goals should give you direction in your training and will build staying power helping you to ride out the down times when you feel you are not reaching other goals. You may miss one goal but if you know that there is another goal that you have to reach then you just have to 'get back on the horse' and carry on.

15. Changing Your Routines

Anything which you do repeatedly will become monotonous, even if it is something you enjoy. The same applies to training routines. To stop yourself becoming bored and potentially giving up on your training program you must vary your routine to keep it interesting.

Not only will you become bored of your routines but if you do the same list of exercises at every session, your muscles will also become used to it and they will stop or slow down in their gains.

Follow some of the ideas below to vary your routine which will help to keep you interested and increase your commitment to your training program.

One way to add variety to your existing program is to simply increase the intensity level of your exercises dramatically. By doing this you will greatly decrease the number of reps you are able to complete for each exercise but it will give your muscles and program a much needed shock. Just do this for a few sessions before returning to your standard level of intensity but it will have done the job.

Rather than do a routine where you exercise all your muscle groups, try concentrating on your upper body for one session and then at the next session, concentrate on your lower body. This will not only allow you to mix up your training but it wall also allow you to target muscles for more intense workouts.

16. Give Your Muscles A Rest

Your muscle need time to rest while they grow. After a heavy workout the muscle do not grow instantly but they require a period of rest while they regenerate. When they do regenerate they will grow bigger and stronger if you have placed enough stress on them.

Not giving your muscles time to rest will actually reduce the amount of growth and reduce any increase in strength. This is why it is a good idea to work muscles on alternative days.

If you exercise all your muscles in each session, it is best to train one day and then rest the next day. If you do want to train every day then you should exercise your upper body on one day and then on the next day, while your upper body is resting from its exertions, you should exercise your lower body. Your lower body would then be rested on the following day which is when you would return to exercising your upper body.

While you are resting, you should make sure that you are taking on enough nutrients to support the growth of your muscles. It is not only while you are exercising that your muscles need energy. Your muscles also need energy to continue growing while they are resting.

17. Increase Number Of Sets

To increase gains in muscle mass and strength you will find that completing multiple sets will have the desired effect.

Being careful not to over exercise, you should complete a set of exercises for a specific muscle then take a short break. The break should only be able a minute long and just enough time for your muscle to recover some of its composure. You would then repeat the same exercise until you could not manage another rep. You will not be able to complete as many reps during the second set as you completed in the first set. This is usual as your muscles will be tired from the first set.

Reaching your maximum intensity in a shorter period of time for the second set will give you the chance to take your muscle to its maximum for the second time in your workout. This is why using multiple sets will help increase muscle mass and strength.

18. Fast And Slow Reps

We have discussed in a previous section about how to kick start your muscles if they stop increasing in size and strength by varying your routine. Another way to give your muscles a kick start is to vary th speed of your reps.

You will have a standard speed which you will complete your exercises in and your muscles will become used to this. Try alternating this by completing really slow sets. Really slow down each execution of an exercise so that you are taking twice or three times as long as normal to complete an exercise.

Slowing down the speed of your reps will place more intensity on the muscle being exercised and you will really be able to feel the difference.

Use these slow reps to also really concentrate on the form of your exercises. Make sure that you are completing them as they should be done. Focus on targeting the actual muscle you are exercising and let your other muscles relax.

Completing slow reps therefore gives you a three fold advantage. Firstly you will be able to load the intensity on the muscle. Secondly you will be giving your muscles some variety. Thirdly you will be able to concentrate on the form of your exercises to make absolutely sure that you are completing each exercise to perfection.

19. Keeping Records

Having records of your progress can be a great motivational tool.

Keeping records from day 1 can show you how far you have come when you look back on these records.

Take photographs of your body from different angles and write down the dates the photos were taken. When you take further photographs at various intervals, possibly at the beginning of each month, you will be able to see very quickly how you are progressing. They can also make it obvious where you need to concentrate so that you can adjust your long term goals to keep your body shape looking balanced.

Along with photographs you should also take measurements as these can give you a more exact record of how muscle sizes are increasing. Measure such as your thighs, waist, chest, neck, arms and keep a date when you take the measurements.

Another record to keep is the size of the weights which you are lifting. You will be surprised at how quickly you can increase the weights which you are lifting and when you start to look back at weights you were lifting just weeks before it will be another reason to spur you on to further success.

20. Do Not Take Risks

Taking risks with training programs should not be done because if you do injure yourself then you will not be able to exercise otherwise you will risk damaging yourself further.

Not only will an injury stop you from training but it will also stop you from carrying out your daily tasks which you take for granted such as going to work, going out shopping, socialising and all the other activities which you enjoy.

You should not hold you breath while exercising as this increases your blood pressure. Make sure you take steady and measured breaths and this will help with your blood pressure and also make sure that you are breathing in enough oxygen to help your muscles perform to their maximum efficiency.

21. Concentrate When Exercising

When you are working out you should be concentrating on the actual exercises. If you are chatting to someone else who may be exercising at the side of you then you risk not completing the reps with the correct form and therefore reducing the effectiveness of the effort which you are putting in to your training program.

If you want to socialise, do this either before or after your training session. When you are training, you should be concentrating on the task in hand. Peak concentration will help you reach your goals much quicker.

Concentrating on the workout routine will also mean that you can get through the program much quicker which means you will then be free to go out socialising sooner than you would if you had been casually chatting to people on the next piece of equipment.

22. Everybody Is Different

Some people are born with genetics which will mean that they can put on masses of bulk while others can train and train without seeing a great deal of increase for their work.

Sometimes you have to accept that you will not have the perfect genetics to build the exact body shape you would like but this is something you will have to accept but then target the exercises which will give greatest benefit.

There are three main body types of genetically determined body structures. These are ectomorphs, mesomorphs and endomorphs.

Ectomorphs are slender in appearance and have difficulty putting on muscle mass.
Endomorphs have thick bones, tend to be heavy and are sometimes fat. They can easily put on muscle mass but find it difficult to lose weight.
Mesomorphs are in between the other body types with moderate bone structures and muscular physiques.

23. Aerobic Exercising

If you want to lose weight then aerobic exercise can be great way to burn fat and also strengthen your cardiovascular system by forcing your heart to work at elevated levels for longer periods of time.

If your training is geared more around building muscle size and strength then aerobic exercising can actually reduce the gains in muscle size and strength.

Aerobic exercising is very beneficial but if you are trying to build muscle it is advisable to limit your aerobic exercise levels to about 1 to 1 ½ hours per week.

There is no reason you should totally abandon aerobic exercising because it does help when body building as it helps to burn off the free fatty acids in the body which results in a more defined, muscular physique.

24. Eat Protein

Protein is incredibly important for muscle growth and should form part of your healthy diet when trying to build your body. There are many different proteins in your body and they are all made either directly or indirectly from the amino acids in the foods and supplements which you eat.

You may see RDA (Recommended Dietary Allowance) levels shown on food packaging and you should pay attention to these important labels. Athletes need much more than the RDA levels when they are burning up the calories during workouts.

Most strength athletes should eat 0.8 grams of protein per pound of body weight per day. Endurance athletes need 0.6 grams per pound of body weight daily. Divide the protein requirement into four or five equal portions to be eaten throughout the day.

To supplement your daily intake of protein while you are training, you may consider protein powders which can help your body take in the required amounts of protein. Many protein powders can easily be mixed with water to give a drink which can quickly be taken while exercising.

25. Carb Choices

Carbohydrates are essential for your body as they are converted to glucose which is the body's preferred source of fuel.

Some carbs are assimilated much more quickly than others and so you should pay attention to which carbs you use. The carbs you should mainly eat are the ones which have a low glycemic index. Examples of carbs with low G.I. are pasta, beans, vegetables and fruits.

An intake of 2 to 3 grams per pound of body weight per day is sufficient for most athletes.

There are many reference books which give a great deal of information about glycemic index levels and you should find one which at least gives you the basics of the foods you are eating so that you can make informed decisions about your dietary intake.

26. Low Fat

You should try and reduce the amounts of fat which you consume if you want a healthy body and you want to improve your results from training.

Not all fats are bad and so you should not try to totally eliminate fat from your diet. Your body needs a small amount of two essential fatty acids every day and these are linoleic acid (omega-3 fatty acid) and linolenic acid (omega-6 fatty acid). Flaxseed oil is an excellent source of both these acids although they are found in smaller amounts in fish and other fatty foods.

If your diet is made up of around 10 to 15 percent fat then that will usually provide enough of these essential fatty acids.

Depending upon your workout program and metabolism levels, greater fat intake may result in body fat accumulation without any corresponding sports benefits.

To limit your exposure to saturated fats you should eat mainly fish, chicken, turkey and egg whites for your protein sources. You should reduce your consumption of beef, pork and egg yolk to a minimum. When buying meat you should buy a very lean cut and trim away all of the visible fat. You should also try and avoid fast food which is generally very high in saturated fats.

27. Eat Well And Often

Your muscles require nutrients on a regular basis if they are expected to grow in size and strength. In order to build muscles you will have to give your muscles the proteins, carbs, fats and micronutrients they need to support the growth process throughout the day.

You should never skip breakfast and also make sure that you eat immediately after your workout routine and then again two hours later.

Instead of the standard 3 meals a day, if you increase to four or five meals a day it will result in a slightly raised metabolic rate too which will help to keep your body fat level under control.

Regular, smaller meals will also help to give your body the nutrients it needs when it needs them rather than two large meals fitted in whenever you can squeeze them in. Being committed and consistent with your meals will pay off in the long run.

28. Balanced Diet

A healthy diet is important but is especially important when you are training as workouts put extra strain on your bodies resources.

You should try and eat a wide variety of health foods to keep your diet varied and interesting.

Make sure you eat lots of fruits and vegetables to give your body a wide variety of essential nutrients to support your muscles while they grow and develop.

Eating the same fruit all the time will become boring and will also limit the different nutrients available to your body. By eating a wide variety of fruits, you will make sure that you have an interesting and enjoyable diet along with supplying your body with everything it needs.

29. Water

One of the essential parts to a healthy diet is water. Many people over look this very important dietary requirement and will be decreasing their gains because of this over sight.

Muscles are made up of up to 70 per cent water and so reducing the amount of water you drink can have dramatic consequences.

Protein synthesis is actually increased when the muscles are fully hydrated which shows how important it is to have plenty of water during the day.

Make sure you eat plenty of foods which have a high water content and you should also drink about 1 ½ to 2 litres of water per day which is about 6 or 8 glasses of water. Taking on water is especially important during the summer when you lose significant amounts of water due to sweating.

30. Be Consistent

Using fad diets or yo-yo dieting actually destroys muscle tissue and so these types of diets should be avoided if it is muscle that you are trying to build.

The best way is to stay lean all year round rather than pilling on the weight only to fast in order to lose the weight again.

You should not starve yourself to lose weight and on the flip side, you should also not over eat either. Controlling your food intake with adequate quantities of protein, carbs and fats will allow your body to build permanent muscle mass without allowing the body to generate fat which would hide your hard-earned gains from your training program.

31. Take A Break

There will always be times when you become bored of your diet while on your training program and to relieve this boredom, sometimes it is useful to allow yourself the opportunity to take a break.

You will not be able to continually take breaks and eat unhealthy foods otherwise you would quickly add body fat and undo all the work you have put in. Taking a break now and then though will give you some motivation that you are allowed some treats when you feel it would help your mood.

Many athletes are incredibly single-minded that they follow strict diets to the letter and will not take a break however this can sometimes be overkill and can ultimately lead to diminished drive and motivation..

Some athletes see Sunday as their 'day-off' and allow themselves some things which they would not generally allow themselves. Do not beat yourself up if you do enjoy some occasional unhealthy options as long as it does not become the norm. Make sure that when you have treated yourself for a while that you are ready to get back into your program with added enthusiasm.

32. Vitamins And Minerals

While you are training, it is essential that your body is given all the nutrients it requires. Vitamins and minerals are essential for good health and peak performance. This is definitely true when you are putting your body under the extreme pressure of a training program.

For those who are not training, it should be easy to obtain all the vitamins and minerals required from a standard well balanced diet. However when you are putting your body under the extreme requirements of a training program your body will require some additional help to take in enough vitamins and minerals to cope.

To make sure that your body has enough of what it needs, try taking multi-vitamins and multi-mineral tablets which will give 100 per cent of the required RDA and these should be taken twice a day to make absolutely sure that you have covered all bases.

Additionally you should also take extra doses of calcium, magnesium along with the antioxidant vitamins C and E.

33. Creatine

Creatine is the most effective sports supplement currently available without a prescription. Your body does naturally produce creatine and it is essential in the role of muscle contraction.

Creatine supplements have been scientifically proven to boost strength and power and so it is ideal for those wanting to improve muscle mass and strength.

Building lean muscle mass is one effect of using creatine supplements and it may also help in protein synthesis.

Take 4 to 12 grams of creatine per day depending on your exercise intensity and muscle mass. This amount of creatine should be divided into two or three doses.

34. Glutamine

Glutamine is an amino acid which plays many vital roles within your body. It will help to reduce the build up of lactic acid which is a by product of exercising. Glutamine will also increase the production of growth hormone which will help to increase muscle mass and helps to permit a more effective training session.

A further advantage of taking glutamine is that it helps to regulate protein synthesis and improves immune system function.

Take 5 grams of glutamine before you start your workout session. Consume 2 to 3 grams on an empty stomach several times a day to maximise the secretion of growth hormone.

35. MSM

MSM has been around for many years but it has only recently been discovered by athletes that there are benefits for those who are training.

It can dramatically reduce the delayed onset of muscle soreness which occurs when pushing your body to the limits with intense exercise.

Start with a dose of 2 grams and slowly increase the dose up to 5 grams over a period of a few weeks. Take two doses on training days, with one dose before you start and the other dose when you have finished your session. A single dose is sufficient on your rest days.

MSM crystals have a bitter taste and so you will probably want to use capsules.

36. Supplements

Supplements may be able to help add extra nutrients, protein and vitamins etc but they are quite expensive. To save money, it is wise to try and get most of your requirements via your diet by carefully choosing what you eat and drink. Supplements should only be used to supplement your diets with things that you think you are lacking from your natural diet.

When buying supplements, you should start by buying the most important ones for your particular needs. It would probably be useful to start by using protein powders. The next supplement you would probably move onto would be creatine. Vitamins and minerals would probably be the next item on your check list. If your budget will still allow it, then it may be now time to move on to using glutamine and MSM.

Whole foods should make up the majority of your diet with supplements only filling in the gaps of where you feel your diet is lacking.

37. Choose Your Time

Different people have different body clocks and you should listen to your when you are deciding your training timetable.

If you are a morning person then you should try and train in the morning. If you work better on an afternoon or in the evening you should push your training sessions to later in the day.

By training when your energy levels are at their peak you ill be able to maximise your intensity and give yourself the best possible chance of the greatest gains in muscle mass and strength. If you tried training when your energy levels are low, you will be more likely to give up sooner and lose out on much of your potential.

38. Stick To The Program

It can be too easy to start and think of missing a training session. This will then turn into missing a couple of sessions. Before too long you will have totally abandoned your training program and not be completing any exercise.

You must stick to the program if you have any hope of making the gains you want. Discipline is very important when you are trying to build your body but it is an essential aspect of your program.

Too much exercise will not allow your body to recover between each training session but you must not use this as an excuse to start missing sessions because too little exercise will mean that your resolve to complete the course will start slipping.

You must try hard to be disciplined with both your exercise program and your diet to achieve maximum results.

39. Create A Balanced Life

Even though you must be disciplined with your training program and your diet, you must also realise that you do have to have a balanced life so that you feel fulfilled.

Work, family and friends add meaning to your life and while you may have to neglect parts of your life if you want to achieve goals in your body building you must make some time to give quality time to these other aspects of your life.

Try and balance all aspects of your life which are important to you so that you feel satisfied and happy. When your life is in balance, you will feel much happier in general and this will help with your commitment and motivation for your training program.

40. Rest

There is definitely such a thing as too much training and this can harm your development. You must make sure that you give your body the time it needs to develop and grow following a training session otherwise muscle mass and strength could actually be reduced.

Your muscles will feel sore after a workout but they should recover within a day. If they are not recovering in a day, in time for the next session, then you are pushing your body too far and you need to listed to what your body is telling you and start to slow down a little.

While your body is resting after a workout session, it may not feel as though your body is doing anything to advance your body building goals but you must understand that the muscles are developing while you let them rest.

41. Sleep

Much of your body's recovery process will take place while you are sleeping which is why making sure you get a good nights sleep is incredibly important.

The greatest release of growth hormone also takes place at night while you are sleeping.

You can not make up for lost sleep and you should try for 7 or 8 hours of sound sleep every night. To help your body with your sleep pattern, try and go to bed at the same time each night.

Sleep is good to help recover from a training session and it is also good because it will rest your body and allow it to prepare for your next training session.

42. Patience

Patience is a virtue. You will not build massive muscles and great strength overnight. It takes time and you should understand that the training sessions are part of a long term plan for your body.

Muscle growth occurs in spurts. You may feel great while your muscles are growing but you must show a great deal of patience when the growth is not as dramatic as it sometimes is at its peak.

Do not become discouraged but simply be patient and understand that if you keep going with your training program, the results will definitely appear.

43. Stress

Stress can reduce your muscle growth and can even stop any growth completely.

The body responds to stress by releasing the catabolic hormone cortical.

Exercising is a great way to relieve stress and anger so you can use it in a positive way by really throwing yourself into your training program to beat the stress and anger which may build up from time to time.

44. Alcohol

Excessive alcohol use can dramatically reduce your gains in muscle mass and strength.

Alcohol reduces the release of growth hormone which is a vital ingredient for muscle growth and strength gains.

Alcohol has also been scientifically shown to shrink the muscle fibres of alcoholics.

If you use alcohol frequently, simply cutting back on your intake will result in a more anabolic environment which will help to promote your gains in muscle mass and strength.

45. Illness

Many athletes resume their maximum intensity workouts as soon as they are over a cold or other illness but these practices will lead to straining your immune system and can actually cause a relapse of the illness which you have just been recovering from.

Some people believe that they can 'sweat it out' when they are suffering from a cold but it will probably cause the illness to last longer as you are not letting your body use its immune system to fully recover. Your body only has so much nutrients to support itself and if you are pushing your body to use these nutrients for training then it will not have sufficient reserves to also combat illness.

Try to ease yourself back into your training program to allow your body to fully recover an in the long run, this will help to stimulate a higher growth rate.

46. Trial And Error

You will make mistakes in your training program and diet choices but this should not be a major problem as long as you are able to learn from these mistakes.

You must experiment with your training program and diets so that you can find the ideal workout and meal plans for you. Everyone is different and so one plan may be right for some people but my not be the best option for yourself. Test lots of different ways and you will also find it more interesting rather than choosing a plan on day 1 and sticking to it forever.

Do not become disheartened if you make some mistakes along the way. This is the only way which will allow you to learn the best way for you and keep you interested.

47. Confidence

A confident attitude will help to increase your mental ability and your physical power.

Instead of continually doubting yourself, make sure that you push forward with strength and conviction.

Confidence is totally different from arrogance. Be confident that you will succeed in attaining your goals and push forward in the knowledge that you are doing your absolute best.

48. Positive Mental Attitude

Building muscle is a very hard task and one of the hardest parts is making sure that you maintain a constructive frame of mind rather than letting yourself become disillusioned.

Make sure you surround yourself with people who will give you positive reinforcement. You do not want people around you saying that you will never make it as that is a sure fire way for you to abandon your goals. Make friends with people who believe in you and people who will tell you that you can achieve anything you set your mind to.

This is a two way street. You should also be positive about other people too. Do not pull down the efforts of other but encourage them to o their best at what they are trying to achieve.

This does not have to be all about training either. Be supportive about the people around you for all their goals and aspirations and they will in turn be supportive with you.

49. Take A Break

Even though you take breaks between training sessions to allow your muscles to recover and grow this is not enough.

You should sometimes take a holiday away from your training to really give your body plenty of time to totally relax.

Exercising in an intensive training program can really take it out of your body and taking a long holiday away from the intense workouts can work wonders for your body and your mental attitude. You should be able to come back from a really relaxing holiday in a really enthusiastic way, ready to really start pushing yourself again.

50. Long Term Goals

Set yourself long term goals which you want to aim towards.

If you set yourself these goals in the distance, you always have something to aim for and it can make sure that you are not always just aiming for short term self-gratification goals.

Enjoy your journey of building your body into a fit and healthy physique. It should be enjoyable even though it will be hard work.

If you have long term goals, you will be able to work harder during your training sessions knowing that you have something worthwhile to aim for in the future.

1 Hour Muscles gives you all the information
you need to achieve a muscular and toned body.

Work out at home without any gym equipment.

Just 20 minutes a day for 3 days a week.

You will be amazed at the results.

Reviews

I really like your "1 Hour Muscles" book. It's fast, it gets right to the point, and it almost turns my laptop into a personal trainer (it's that good!)
Thank you for giving people such an easy way to build muscle mass. Just "Rule 1" was worth the price of the book for me, because probably over the last three to four months I've been driving 15-20 minutes three times a week to the nearest gym, and my girlfriend hasn't even said anything yet about all the time I've spent working out. Turns out after reading "Rule 1" I know why I have had only slight results to speak of so far. I'm really excited about doing your workout and quite possibly no longer using the gym, because "1 Hour Muscles" makes that unnecessary.
Dan Klatt

I've only just stopped aching enough to type after following the exercises. They were easy enough to do in the office, and I did them in my lunch hour with my colleagues. I can see how I will benefit from each exercise and even after a few days can feel a difference.
I can't wait for summer now, as I'll be able to put all the other guys on the beach to shame!
David Chamberlain

I have read "1 Hour Muscle" twice and I must say it changed the way I work out. I felt a good progress just by reading the program's rules and applying them to my workout.
This book offers you a complete and easy to follow training program that should be doable for everyone. But for me, the best part is the workout rules, those rules work and I suggest you use them.
You may want to read this book even if you love your current training program, it can add great value
D.H.Mason

www.ingramcontent.com/pod-product-compliance
Lightning Source LLC
Chambersburg PA
CBHW051956280526
45793CB00005B/741

9 781442 186606